Winning Strategies for Successful Aging

Date: 3/13/13

YALE UNIVERSITY PRESS HEALTH & WELLNESS

A Yale University Press Health & Wellness book is an authoritative, accessible source of information on a health-related topic. It may provide guidance to help you lead a healthy life, examine your treatment options for a specific condition or disease, situate a healthcare issue in the context of your life as a whole, or address questions or concerns that linger after visits to your healthcare provider.

For a complete list of titles in this series, please consult yalebooks.com.

Winning Strategies for Successful Aging

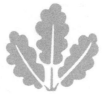

Eric Pfeiffer, M.D.

Yale UNIVERSITY PRESS
New Haven & London

The information and suggestions contained in this book are not intended to replace the services of your physician or caregiver. Because each person and each medical situation is unique, you should consult your own physician to get answers to your personal questions, to evaluate any symptoms you may have, or to receive suggestions for appropriate medications.

The authors have attempted to make this book as accurate and up to date as possible, but it may nevertheless contain errors, omissions, or material that is out of date at the time you read it. Neither the authors nor the publisher has any legal responsibility or liability for errors, omissions, out-of-date material, or the reader's application of the medical information or advice contained in this book.

Published on the foundation established in memory of William Chauncey Williams of the Class of 1822, Yale Medical School, and of William Cook Williams of the Class of 1850, Yale Medical School.

Published with assistance from the foundation established in memory of Calvin Chapin of the Class of 1788, Yale College.

Yale University Press books may be purchased in quantity for educational, business, or promotional use. For information, please e-mail sales.press@yale.edu (U.S. office) or sales@ yaleup.co.uk (U.K. office).

Designed by James J. Johnson.
Set in Swift type by Integrated Publishing Solutions.
Printed in the United States of America.

Library of Congress Cataloging-in-Publication Data
Pfeiffer, Eric, 1935–
Winning strategies for successful aging / Eric Pfeiffer.
p. cm.
Includes index.
ISBN 978-0-300-18402-0 (pbk. : alk. paper)
1. Older people—Health and hygiene.   2. Older people—Mental health.
3. Self-care, Health.   I. Title.
RA777.6P44 2012
613'.0438—dc23   2012019766

A catalogue record for this book is available from the British Library.

This paper meets the requirements of ANSI/NISO Z39.48–1992 (Permanence of Paper).

10 9 8 7 6 5 4 3 2 1

To the many patients, family members, friends,
and acquaintances who
through the power of their example
have taught me the many ways of
aging successfully

Contents

CONTENTS

Foreword

George E. Vaillant, M.D.

Eric Pfeiffer has written a useful, Dr. Spock–like handbook for growing old, a book that can be kept in easy reach and referred to whenever you feel you need useful facts or advice.

However, he has written much more than that: he has written a very wise book. When you begin to read this book, start with the last chapters—where the "music" lives. By reading Chapters 12 through 15 first, you can learn to trust that the author has traveled the path that you are traveling with compassion and deep understanding, and that you can trust the good advice of the earlier chapters.

Eric Pfeiffer is ideally suited to write this book. I have been following his career as a friend and as a student for 45 years, so I know a little about what I am promising the reader. Eric had written a textbook of psychiatry by the time he finished residency. In other words, he was not satisfied with just learning a field, but he wished to become its master.

Equally important, by the time Pfeiffer finished medical school he had already published his first book of poetry—and not with a vanity press. He understood the *heart* of medicine as well as the facts. Then for the next 45 years Eric has been a gerontologist as a researcher, as a practitioner, and as an administrator. *Winning Strategies for Successful Aging* is what you would expect from a polymath, a poet, and a lifelong competitor. It is a very wise book on how to succeed in aging.

Chapter 12 directs elders to turn inward after retirement and to remember that they have souls as well as bodies. Spend some time remembering who, as a teenager, you wanted to become; ask yourself what animal you would like to be. And to quote Pfeiffer, "Being in touch with one's soul is what the poet Wallace Stevens said was 'finding what will suffice.' It allows us to live in a harmonious relationship with all of nature and the creatures in it, including all of humanity." Chapter 13 reminds us that it is just as exciting and romantic to get married at age 75 as at 21—a surprising and very useful lesson.

Chapter 14 helps remind us that the key to happiness is to remember that life is not all about us. To keep it, you have to give it away. Pfeiffer offers a memorable quote from a media commentator: "The way we get to live forever is through memories stored in the hearts and souls of those whose lives we touch." Pfeiffer also reminds us that in old age one of the greatest gifts that we can give ourselves is to forgive those who have "trespassed" against us. Finally, in Chapter 15, Pfeiffer very gently holds us, as a mother might, while he helps us to bring into consciousness the fact that the death rate is still one per person and we damned well better plan for our death.

Introduction

DEAR READER: Welcome to *Winning Strategies for Successful Aging*. I am assuming that either you are a baby boomer, approaching the threshold of senior citizenship and trying to prepare for it, or that you have already passed age 65 and are looking to improve your ongoing aging experience. Or perhaps you are the adult child of aging parents who wants to better understand your father's and mother's aging experiences. Good for you, for being concerned about their success. Maybe, after you have learned all that you can from this guide, you can pass this book on to your parents for their possible enjoyment and enlightenment. They will be pleased that you cared, and they may be surprised to find how much of this book applies directly to them. Even if you don't share this book with them, they will be delighted at how much you know and understand about their aging experience.

In any case, I am very glad you are here, and I welcome you to what promises to be an exciting journey. Throughout this book I will be addressing you directly as though we were sitting together in a comfortable living room, or in a study, or out on your back porch.

This book will teach you how *you can control and direct* your own aging. You will discover approaches to help you reach your desired destination, so that you can free yourself of many of the fears you may have had about growing older. And you will discover that senior citizenship not only is manageable but can be the pinnacle of your well-lived life. In this book you will receive step-by-step advice on how to negotiate all the major areas of your aging experience. You will learn what successful aging is and how to achieve it. You will learn that you have years and years left to live in which to enjoy yourself and to accomplish things you have had to postpone until now. You will learn about the joy of place: choosing a place to live that is ideally suited to your wants and needs in retirement. You will learn how you can become the older person you want to be. You will understand the importance of your social connections, including your spouse but also your much larger social network. I will talk about how to hold on to your physical health, your mental health, and your wealth, and how to maintain your brain. You will learn the importance of exercise. You will learn how to fight to maintain your independence and how to plan to receive care if and when you need it. You will learn about your rich inner mental and psychological life, your spirituality, and your sexuality. A few very personal thoughts—actually, personal *secrets*—of successful aging follow; thoughts and ideas that have lit my way and that may be of some interest to you as well. Finally, an extensive appendix deals with a variety of issues that may crop up as you age.

Winning Strategies for Successful Aging is based on my experience as a psychiatrist and a gerontologist. For some 12 years I was a member of the Duke University Center for the Study of Aging in Durham, North Carolina, and for more than 30 years I served as the Founding Director of the Suncoast Alzheimer's and Gerontology Center at the College of Medicine at the University of South Florida in Tampa. In these positions I had the opportunity to treat and to study thousands of older people and their loved ones as they navigated this critical phase of their lives. I learned from them and from my research what works and what doesn't work. This is my attempt to distill that knowledge and make it available to you. I want this to be a conversation between you and me that is useful, practical, and understandable, so that you can make this phase of your life enjoyable, successful, and relatively trouble-free.

From time to time throughout the book I have included a poem to emphasize or to illustrate a particular issue. All the poems included here are mine, and they are all drawn from a volume of poetry published in 2010, *Under One Roof,* which is cited in the "About the Author" section of this book. If you are not into poetry, which I can certainly understand, you can skip the poems. Or, taken in context, they may open another window to your own aging experience.

Chapter 1

You Have a Whole Generation of Life Left to Live— Prepare Accordingly

OST PEOPLE want to live a long life. They want to become wiser, smarter, happier, and more serene as they age. Never has this been truer than for the baby boomer generation. As a member of that generation you should know that you are on the forefront of a new way of experiencing the later years. Until recently, when people reached retirement or passed the 65-year mark, they had a relatively short span of life remaining. But no more! *You can't count on dying any time soon!* Your generation can expect to live 10, 15, 20, 25, or even 30 more years after crossing the milestone of your 65th birthday. You may even become a *centenarian!* In short, *you have a whole generation of life left to live.* What does that mean?

It means you need to prepare accordingly. And that is the exact purpose of this book: to help you prepare for this next phase of your life—a phase that may be as long as the time from infancy to full adulthood. Look back on that period of your life: what a period of growth it was, what changes occurred, and what an adventure it was. And so it will be with this coming period of your life, if you make it so, if you take an active role in *directing* your own aging. *You* are in charge, and *you* can have the time of your life in making this *the best time of your life*. Your generation can experience aging like no other group of individuals before you. You have the skills and the tools and the will for planning and preparing to accomplish these goals.

Write Down Your Goals and Strategies

You can set goals for yourself—large and numerous goals that are beyond anything you ever dreamed of. Once you think of the coming years as a whole generation of life left to live, it becomes clear that you need to develop goals and strategies to accomplish those goals that are commensurate with your vision. These goals need to be written down and must include detailed strategies in each of the areas that are discussed in this book: where to live, what to do, who to be, what kind of a social network you want to have. You need goals related to your physical health, to your mental health, and to your finances. You need goals related to your spiritual self, your sexuality, and your charitable activities.

The likelihood of achieving a goal increases dramatically when you have written goals, accompanied by written strategies, and by a plan for measuring how far you have come toward achieving your goals. To make it even more likely that you achieve your goals, *journal your journey;* that is, write down in a private journal, for your eyes only, how far you have come and what obstacles you may have encountered. A brief summary appears at the end of each chapter from here on in. You may want to use these summaries as a guide to measure how you are doing. If it all turns out to be really interesting, you could even make it into a memoir and publish it, for your children and grandchildren, or even for the world at large.

You Can Amend Your Goals and Your Strategies

You will have ample opportunity to amend your goals and your strategies. If something doesn't work out, or if something doesn't satisfy, you can set new goals and develop new strategies. From here on out there is no such thing as failure. If you don't like the results, change your goals and change your strategies. You might even find yourself saying, Why didn't I think of this before? Why didn't I run my whole life like this? Never mind, don't bother to look back. Just do it from here on forward. Start from where you are. A journey of a thousand miles begins with a *single* step; it begins with a decision; it begins from where you are *now*.

Old Age Is Not for Sissies, and You Are No Sissy

You may have heard it said that "old age is not for sissies," and "don't go out there without your helmet on." There is considerable truth in these assertions. Nor is old age necessarily automatically "golden," unless you actively work to make it so. Old age is also called "a season of loss" as friends and relatives die, as one's job identity disappears, and physical strength wanes. In this book you will learn how best to respond to these losses, and to the many other challenges that you may face. But you will also find that as you grow older, new opportunities and new insights will emerge, and along with everything else an understanding that only a really long life can provide. So get ready for an exciting journey. Get ready for successful aging.

CHAPTER SUMMARY

- You have a whole generation of life left to live.
- You can't count on dying any time soon.
- Make this the best time of your life.
- Have written goals and written strategies.
- Journal your journey.
- You can amend your goals and your strategies.
- Old age is not for sissies, and you're no sissy.
- Insist on aging successfully.

Chapter 2

Understand What Successful Aging Is, and Then Plan to Do It

What Is Successful Aging, and Is It Possible to Age Successfully?

SUCCESSFUL AGING is living the life *you* have envisioned—with gusto, energy, and enjoyment. It means a life filled with activities that are meaningful to you; a life filled with friendships and loving relationships, as well as with challenges that you will address and manage so they don't become unbearable, ongoing problems.

Is such successful aging possible? Definitely. We each have seen many successfully aging individuals among family members, friends, and acquaintances. We each know individuals who are "going great guns" at 80, 85, and even at 90 years old. A number of public figures have shown what can still be accomplished in later life. Grandma Moses took up a career in painting when she was in her 70s; Ruth Rothfarb ran her first marathon when she was 80; Helen Santmyer published her first novel, a best-seller, when she was in her 80s; Pablo Casals gave concerts on his cello until he was well into his 90s; Picasso continued to paint in his 90s. The actress Angela Lansbury, at age 83, took on a new role on Broadway in Noel Coward's play *Blythe Spirit*. A few years back, the *St. Petersburg Times* published an article titled "80 Over 80," featuring 80 individuals who remained influential in their ninth decade and beyond; among the list were Alan Greenspan, economist, age 90; Carl Reiner, actor, writer, and director, age 87; Pete Seeger, folk singer, age 90; Barbara Walters, journalist and media personality, age 80; George H. W. Bush, 41st president of the United States; I. M. Pei, prize-winning architect, age 92; Maya Angelou, poet and civil rights activist, age 81; Helen Thomas, journalist, age 89; Dave Brubeck, jazz pianist, age 88; Henry Kissinger, former secretary of state, age 86; Jack LaLanne, exercise guru, age 95; Cloris Leachman, Oscar-winning actress, age 83; and many others. Many of them are still going strong. Numerous patients of mine met and married in their late 80s and are very much enjoying their new life together. Thus, successful aging is possible, but it is by no means the norm. It doesn't just happen; it must be planned for and achieved.

Can successful aging be learned? Can it be taught? Can it be fostered and promoted? Again, the answer to all of these questions is definitely "yes." You can learn from other successfully aging persons. You will read about some of their experiences and their strategies. And be assured that in order to age successfully you don't have to do anything spectacular or something that makes the evening news or the Guinness Book of World Records. All you need to do is to map out *your* plan, follow that plan, and reach *your* goals for *your* life.

From time to time in this book I share brief case histories from my years of practice with older patients that illustrate a particular point. Accordingly, I want to tell you about one remarkable lady who came to me for help during my days at Duke University. In the process of my trying to help her, I benefited greatly from what she taught me. And you may be able to benefit from her experience as well.

At age 71 Aileen, recently widowed, contemplated what lay ahead for her. In her grief over her beloved husband she envisioned a rather bleak future for herself, and on several occasions seriously considered committing suicide. She mentioned this to her doctor, who was not particularly alarmed and who did not refer her for help.

But as she was about to walk into a lake to drown herself she was suddenly hit by the realization that what she was about to do was totally inconsistent with the life she had lived until then. She turned around and went to see a psychiatrist instead.

The psychiatrist recognized that Aileen was depressed and began treatment immediately, with good results. After six months of intensive interactive psychotherapy and the use of antidepressant medication, Aileen recovered from her depression. She went back to her psychiatrist to report that she had returned to her usual self. She was grateful for the help she had received. Then she shared with him some insights she had gained after coming through the deep valley of depression. She said: "I've been through a lot, but I am okay now. I like where I live, I know who I am, and I am not alone." The psychiatrist was impressed. He realized that he had just heard about the most succinct definition of successful aging. He would remember this phrase for a very long time, and maybe, someday, write a book about it. *Winning Strategies for Successful Aging* is that book.

Incidentally, this lady went on to live an active and enjoyable life until she was 104 years old. She died peacefully only after outlasting a good friend with whom she had had a life-long rivalry and who died at a mere 103. How wrong her doctor had been to ignore her symptoms! She truly demonstrated the fact that many older persons still have a whole generation of life left to live. At one point she even considered marrying again, but then she decided that her relationships with her friends and extended family were enough. She and I became friends and visited with each other from time to time. Her life was full of adventures, and even though she encountered a few additional problems in her later years, she never became depressed again. To this day I am grateful to Aileen for what she taught me. When she had said, "I like where I live, I know who I am, and I am not alone," she had, in fact, described successful aging.

Here's another story, one that is more commonplace, and one you might be able to relate to more easily.

Jack and Jackie were workaholics. Jack ran a construction company that built houses, restaurants, banks, and a few small apartment complexes. Jack had designed and built his own home in a large city where he and his wife lived comfortably for the past ten years. Jackie taught school for the past 30 years, mostly to children from ages six to ten. She was very effective in relating to these children, instilling the love of learning in them rather than simply teaching facts.

Now Jack and Jackie were both 65 and suddenly faced with what to do in their upcoming retirement. Neither of them had any hobbies or significant circle of friends other than work-related associates. As a business owner, Jack had no company pension on which to live, and Jackie's pension consisted of a small amount of money she received from the non-profit school where she had taught. What to do? For a year or so they were quite puzzled. He took on a few relatively small construction projects but really wanted to stop working. She took on a few church-related teaching activities, more to pass the time of day rather than as a money-earning activity or as a real commitment. For approximately a year they visited various retirement communities. They were looking for a community in which the cost of living was lower, and where there were ample activities available and they could develop a new social circle.

Then they heard about a new retirement community just an hour away where all the houses were brand new, and real estate costs were a fraction of what they were in the city where they now lived. This community offered a full range of scheduled activities every day; there were multiple golf courses, and much of the local traffic was done by golf cart rather than automobile. Medical care was readily available. They placed their home on the market, and as soon as it had sold at a good price they purchased a much smaller home in the new retirement community. They invested the money that was freed up into a single-premium annuity payable over both of their lives, and they moved to a whole new lifestyle.

On returning to visit their former neighbors, both Jack and Jackie reported that they were happier than they had ever been in the large city. They had made many new friends in the various activities they each had signed up for. He discovered that he had considerable talent in painting, both with watercolors and acrylics. She took several exercise classes, played mah-jongg on a regular basis, and found a new church with congenial parishioners that had come from all over the United States. The telephone, Internet, and mail correspondence kept them in frequent contact with their extended family. Each of their children visited with them to see where their parents had landed, and they could travel from here to anywhere in the country. They took their first trip to Europe and visited England and France, finding each exciting and totally different from one another. They each felt like they were on a second honeymoon together, affirming time and again that they had made the right decision.

There can be no doubt that successful aging is possible, that it takes many forms, and that it has many faces. One thing is clear, however, and that is that it must satisfy the individual. The case of Jack and Jackie touches on another very interesting issue related to successful aging: Should the pursuit of *happiness* itself be a specific goal in trying to achieve successful aging? My own view is that while one can seek pleasure from a specific activity—be it a great meal, a wonderful vacation, the pleasure of getting a new car, and so on—a direct search for "happiness" is not likely to bear fruit. Rather, as in the case of Jack and Jackie, it may be best to pursue successful aging in its broadest terms, seeking to live a fully realized life, and let happiness emerge as a warmly welcomed side effect of a well-lived life.

CHAPTER SUMMARY

- Successful aging can be learned.
- Successfully aging persons most often like where they live, they know who they are, and they are not alone.
- Search your mind for successfully aging persons you have known, heard of, or read about, and consider emulating them in your own life.
- A direct search for happiness as such is not recommended; rather, let happiness emerge as a welcomed side effect of a well-lived life.

Chapter 3

Choose Your Ideal Place to Live

AS I LOOK out the window at the sun-drenched greenery of my front yard in the morning, I take enormous pleasure in the rich display of light and colors. In the afternoon, when I walk down my street to the Bayshore, a linear park in my neighborhood, I relish the dappled shade that the live oaks cast over the houses and lawns as I greet my neighbors on their front porches. I watch with pleasure the ripple of the gentle breezes on the waters of the bay, and marvel at the herons and gulls. When I sit on my back porch in the evening, I admire the way sunset colors light up the palms and the tangerine trees as I listen to the muffled roar of traffic from the nearby boulevard. It all makes me feel relaxed and fulfilled. In short, I love where I live.

It is important to choose a place to live in retirement with surroundings that will support you and give you daily pleasure. Choosing wisely where to live in retirement will reward you for years and years to come. What makes this time of your life different from all the other times in your life is that *you are now totally portable;* that is, you can now *live anywhere in the world,* unrestricted by job commitments, by college careers, or by where you happen to have been born. You can now find your ideal place to live.

One Possibility: Staying Put

In finding your ideal place to live, there are a lot of things to be considered: climate, transportation, communications, social connections, and available services, among others. But before you decide to pull up stakes and move to some far-off place about which you know very little, first consider retiring in your hometown.

There are many advantages to retiring in your hometown. First of all, you know the territory. You have roots and connections there. You know where everything is: grocery stores, drug stores, churches, doctor's offices, movies, etc. You are familiar with the politics of the place, its newspapers, its sports teams, and so on. You have many friends and acquaintances that provide a social support system. You may have children and grandchildren living there with whom you want to stay close. And you know the climate; you know whether it suits you or not. Moreover, retiring in your own hometown means *you don't have to move.* As well, you avoid the cost of moving.

Very significantly, moving brings with it its own peculiar problems. Personally, moving for me has always been an upsetting experience, even when I was a youngster.

Moving

Disassembled, the moving boxes
gape, or bulge, in every room,
witnessing change. They remind me:
Tenant, I am yet trespasser.
Windows, like sunken eyes,
walls, like blank hostile faces,
stare at me and implore:
Be gone, migrant-vagrant.
Doors open, to let me go.
On the stairs, dissolute
among boxes, I sit.
Moving unhinges me.

Try Something New

On the other hand, you may not like the climate where you live; or you may be tired of some other aspects of your present community; or your children may have moved away and you want to be closer to them; or you may just want to try something new. Your choices are wide open. As I have said, *you are now portable.*

One good way to start thinking about where to live in retirement is to return to some of the places you have visited and have enjoyed during business trips, family visits, or vacations. You may have *always* wanted to live in Florida, or California, or Arizona, or Hawaii, or still other popular vacation or retirement destinations. You might even want to live in Europe, or someplace in South America, or in still more exotic climates or locations. The choice is now yours. You can *scout out* the possible new locations by going there for a few days, or a few weeks, or even for a few months, before making a final decision. It may be of interest to you that hardly anyone ever moves further north in retirement; if people move for their retirement, they are far more likely to move south. This is true not only in America, but in Europe as well. It seems a warmer climate suits us better as we get older.

Apart from geography and climate, there are many other choices for you to consider: Do you want to continue to live entirely independently, or do you want to live in a retirement community? Do you want to live in a freestanding home or in a condominium or townhouse? Do you want to move in with relatives, or have relatives move in with you? There are a lot of issues to consider. So let's deal with these one at a time.

Do You Want to Live Independently or Live in a Retirement Community?

Do you want to continue to live "free range," that is, entirely independently, or do you want to take advantage of some of the benefits that retirement communities have to offer? In a retirement community, many of the obligations you have had while living independently will be taken over for you. You don't have to mow the grass, clean the gutters, fix the roof, paint the house—inside or out, or do other chores that you might want to ditch. You may not even have to cook for yourself anymore, opting instead to enjoy meals provided by a facility, maybe once a day or up to three times a day. And you won't want for company. Plenty of other people will be available with whom you can interact. *You* can decide whether this is what you want. Many retirement communities also offer additional levels of care, such as nursing assistance, in case you should develop a condition that might limit your mobility and for which you might require occasional or daily help (more about this in Chapter 11).

Do You Want to Live in a Condominium or Town House?

Somewhere in between living in a retirement community and living totally independently is condominium living. All the physical chores and external upkeep of your residence and the grounds are taken care of for you. In addition, many condominium facilities have amenities such as swimming pools, gyms, clubhouses, and so on, that are not available to those who live in independent homes. But condominium living is not for everyone. One businessman who moved from a rambling home and waterfront yard to a condominium grumbled about the move: "It's like living in a goddamn motel," he said. He hated the proximity of other people around his unit, and the fact that he felt he had to be dressed up as if for company most of the time.

Should You Move In with Relatives or Have Relatives Move In with You?

You may be invited to "move in with us," by children or other relatives. This (almost) always comes from a sense of love and affection from those issuing the invitation, so you should certainly give it serious consideration. But living with children or other relatives may have downsides that you must also consider. You must make clear your own expectations and those of your relatives. To what extent will you have privacy? Who will prepare meals, and do the dishes? Will you be expected to do some babysitting? What will be the financial arrangements? If all of these things can be worked out to your mutual satisfaction, then you may wish to proceed.

Make Sure Your Ideal Place Is
Ideal for Your Partner, Too

If you are married or living in a committed relationship, the choice of where to live is a two-person decision that needs to satisfy both of your wants and needs. You and your partner may disagree about the importance of this or that aspect of the choice. For this reason, it's important that you explore these choices together. You should consider enough possibilities that an agreement, or at least a happy compromise, can be reached. It is best to eliminate choices that are totally unsatisfactory for one or the other of you. The goodwill and give-and-take that the two of you have established throughout your relationship will come into play in this decision as well.

> John and Linda lived in Rochester, New York. His job with Eastman Kodak had kept him there all during his working years, but the cold winters were getting him down. He wanted to move south—way south. Linda, on the other hand, enjoyed her friends and social connections in Rochester and was reluctant to move. So, they started taking trips together to explore their options, first to North Carolina, then to the Georgia coast. Finally they settled on the west coast of Florida. Linda quickly made new friends, John loved the fishing and the warm weather, and they never looked back, except to occasionally visit what had been home for them for a long time.

Choose Well So That You Only Have to Move Once

One final bit of advice on choosing where to live in retirement: Take your time in making this decision.

Find out all you can about the new place. Meet some of the people who live there. Visit some of the local facilities and amenities. Does the place have tennis, golf, libraries, shopping, etc. to suit your needs? It is so important that you find "joy of place." And you want to get it right the first time. It is not a decision you want to have to make over and over.

CHAPTER SUMMARY

- Where you live influences how you act and feel every day of your life.
- You are now portable. Find your ideal place to live.
- Consider retiring in your hometown.
- You may just want to try something new.
- Do you want to live independently or in a retirement community?
- Do you want to live in a condominium or town house?
- Do you want to move in with relatives or have relatives move in with you?
- Make sure your ideal place is ideal for both you and your partner.
- Choose well so that you only have to move once, or not at all.

Chapter 4

Know Who You Are—and *Do* Something

YOU ARE the main character in this drama called "the rest of your life." But you are now in a whole new phase of your life. You can choose who you want to be and what you want to do in the next 10, 20, perhaps even 30 years of your life. Of course, you will first and foremost want to *be yourself,* the person you have always been, but with a few new wrinkles (pun intended). Now you can choose to add new dimensions to your identity. You can choose to add new activities to your list of what you've already done.

Be Yourself

The opportunity to add these new dimensions and activities to your life is triggered when you drop some of your former identity's activities and aspects as you enter this new phase of your life. If you have been in the workforce, retiring sheds your work identity as well as your work-related activities. You are no longer professor of English, practicing physician, lawyer, teacher, minister, or accountant. If you have not been in the workforce but your spouse or partner has, your identity and activities will change as well when your other half is no longer working. Of course you are still the same person with the same personality you have always been, but now you can add fresh, new dimensions and facets to your life.

What Are Some of the Building Blocks for a Changed Identity?

You might find the building blocks of a new identity hidden within yourself. Or you might look to the outside world for models of who you want to be over the next many years. As mentioned before, the amount of time for which you are planning could be quite extensive! Start by looking within yourself. When you were an adolescent, what did you want to be when you grew up? A mail carrier, a teacher, a politician, a gardener, or president? And when you were working at your job, didn't you sometimes think about a more ideal job than the one you actually had? What was your "dream job"? Was it to be a captain of a pleasure boat, the owner of your own company, a world traveler, a painter, or a writer? When I was an adolescent I wanted to be so many things: a baseball player, a writer, a gardener, a business executive making millions of dollars. As a grown man, I sometimes dreamed of being a bartender, an actor, or the owner of a professional football team. Well, now I do some of those things. I write, and I garden, both of which are very satisfying to me.

What about you? Indulge your fantasy! Didn't you sometimes think: "Wouldn't it be great if I could . . . ?" Well, now you can. You can add color to whatever picture of yourself you have. You can add new facets. You can flesh out one or more dimensions of the person you already are.

In addition to looking inward to your own wishes and dreams, you can also turn outward and look at models in real life or even in fiction that you might wish to emulate: a favorite friend or relative, a character in a play or a movie, someone whose autobiography you have read. You can model yourself after them. You can acquire greater perspective, more tranquility, more peace, or perhaps more excitement than you have had in your life until now. (I explore these issues still further in Chapter 12.)

What Are You Going To Do in Retirement?

"What are you going to do in retirement?" That is the most frequently asked question of people who are about to retire. I know. I was asked innumerable times by friends, colleagues, and family members, and it always made me vaguely uncomfortable. It was as if I was supposed to come up with the "right" answer, or a single answer. I usually responded, "I don't know" or "nothing." But these answers didn't satisfy anyone, including myself. So I began to say that I guessed I would have to figure it out, and that gave me some breathing room. But I knew that eventually I had to address the question in earnest and come up with some real answers for myself.

I began by saying I would write five books. That shut people up pretty quickly. "Five books?" they would say, in astonishment. And I would tell them about the books I was going to write. Well, to date I have published three of the five books I was going to write: First, the book that you are now reading, *Winning Strategies for Successful Aging.* Second, another consumer health book titled *The Art of Caregiving in Alzheimer's Disease,* and third, a book of poems titled *Under One Roof.* There are two further books I am still working on, a somewhat philosophical book titled *Thoughts,* and finally a novel with the somewhat provocative title, *You Are All Sh!&heads!* So these are some of my choices of what to do. What about you?

The question of what to do in retirement is certainly not a simple one. First of all, you are going to be doing many things, not just one, including a good bit of "doing nothing." But that will only get you so far. You will need to generate a more complete answer.

Keep Doing What You Have Been Doing

Again, as with the decision on where to live, you should first consider doing what you have been doing up till now, if that has been satisfying to you. That is, you could continue to work at your job or your profession, but in a much reduced fashion, such as by working part- time, taking only occasional assignments, and so on. Or you could do some variation of what you have been doing, such as "consulting" in the field of your expertise. There are many variations of this consulting work. You could pursue it as a business, or as an occasional hobby, or anything in between. But the idea has considerable merit. You can get paid for consulting, you can stay in contact with people in your field, and there are other benefits too numerous to mention.

Another way of staying active and involved is by doing volunteer work in your area of expertise. This might include providing your services at no cost to those who are not able to afford them, or mentoring younger people in your field. You will be paid in gratitude, not money, and in knowing that you are being of service to someone else.

Start Something Brand New

Whether you're retiring or have never been in the workforce, you can start something brand new. Of course you could also do volunteer work in a totally new arena: volunteering at your local hospital, school, church, or synagogue. Or you might want to deliver Meals on Wheels, drive shut-ins to their doctor's offices, or serve on community boards. All you need to do is to say: "How can I help?" and there will be many people who will respond to your offer. You might learn some new skills in the process, have entirely new experiences, and meet entirely new people from segments of our society other than the one you have been a part of most of your life. It might be an incentive to learn a new language, or simply to gain a new perspective by looking at the world through another set of eyes. You might wish to talk to people already doing volunteer work to learn what they are gaining from their activities.

Yet another approach to deciding what to do in retirement is to think about the things you have always wanted to do but had to postpone because of your other obligations. You might want to learn new things you never had time to do before: to paint; to write poetry; to write an autobiography; to start a new business; to dance; or to play golf. Start or join a book club? Learn to dance? Learn to use the computer, and e-mail, and a digital camera, so you can mail pictures to all of your friends and relatives? Get a smart phone? Play the stock market (but only with your play money, not the money that is funding your retirement)? Go back to college, or finish an abandoned education? Or even go to college for the first time? Many colleges and universities offer free courses for senior citizens on a space-available basis. And you can combine any number of these activities. So let your mind roam free: What would intrigue you? What would be fun to do or to be? There are few limitations; there are only a few obstacles. What you have to do is make a decision, and then try to implement that decision. If you don't like what you started, you can quit. You can change directions and start all over again. What is to stop you?

Up to now I have primarily covered things that people might wish to do after retiring from a job or a profession. But maybe you are among the many who were not formally in the work force (don't ever say to a housewife that she didn't work!). You might now wish to turn your hands or mind or both in a totally new direction. Again, think about what you have always wanted to do. In addition to all the activities listed in the previous paragraph, you could do any or all of the following: Learn to fly a plane? Take a master baking or cooking class? Join a hiking club for seniors? Train guide dogs for the handicapped? Work with returning war veterans to help them find jobs? Learn calligraphy? Take a course in bookbinding (perhaps you could make a book for your family)? Join a bird watching group? Volunteer to teach reading at the public library? Look around you—the opportunities are endless.

Learn a New Skill

Every phase of life requires new skills. Nothing enhances your life experience as much as learning something new: a new language, a new dance step, a new exercise routine, a new investment strategy, reading about people whom you have long admired. The fastest way to learn is by modeling yourself after someone else who speaks another language, who dances a different step, or who reads different books from what you have read so far.

Teach What You Know

While learning a new skill has considerable merit, another idea for something to do in your retirement is almost the exact opposite of learning something new: It is to *teach what you know.* Many of you have amassed knowledge and skills that are well worth passing on to a new generation. Depending on your particular experience and activities, you might want to teach art, calligraphy, music, investment skills, or any number of other skills that a younger person might well wish to acquire. The list of things you could teach is potentially endless. You could teach through your local high school or university, the YMCA, your local library, or your church or synagogue. It is wonderfully rewarding to see young people pick up and cherish skills that you have or things that you know.

Write Your Autobiography

It has been said that "a life worth living is a life worth recording." Writing your autobiography or memoir is one activity that can keep you going for as long as you live, as you will be adding new chapters to your life as you write. At every turn you will discover new facets of the person you thought you knew (i.e., yourself), and you will come to new conclusions and have an entirely new view of the life you have lived.

If you don't know how to get started, or if the task seems too daunting, read the autobiographies of people you admire or are curious about. Your local library is full of memoirs and autobiographies. Another way to get going is to start or to join a memoir-writing group. You could ask about such a group at your local library, or you might consider starting such a group by posting a note inviting others to join you. In the process you will learn a tremendous amount about the lives of other people. Who knows, you might even want to publish your memoirs and become a best-selling author.

Travel the World

Ah, and then there is travel. Some of you have done some traveling as part of your business or your professional life. For the most part that would have been obligatory travel—someone else may have determined your destination, the duration, and the limitations of your travel experience. Now you can go anywhere in the world, for as long as you'd like, by whatever means of travel you choose. You have never had the leisure before to travel by car across country, because you simply could not afford to take that much time.

Is travel expensive? It can be. But you can figure out what you can afford. Here are a few hints that will reduce the cost of travel. You can plan well in advance, and you can travel with groups at group rates. Find out about Road Scholar (formerly known as Exploritas and Elderhostel), which provides travel in groups to interesting destinations, with inexpensive lodging provided. Also, take advantage of the many venues that provide specially discounted rates for senior citizens. These rates may apply to airfare, cruises, theater tickets, and many more activities.

Google the World

Here is another whole new world that can open for you at the click of a button—a computer button, specifically. The amount of information that is available on the Internet is truly astonishing. Search engines such as Google, Yahoo, Bing, Ask, and Dogpile, among others, are truly encyclopedic in what they can provide: you can track down quotes, song lyrics, historical information, event schedules, airline and cruise schedules, price comparisons, and much, much more.

Google yourself, your friends, your favorite author or actor or other celebrity. Many of these individuals have blogs where you can interact with them, ask questions, make suggestions, and so forth. You probably already have a computer, but if you don't, this is the time to acquire a personal computer or a laptop. If you don't own a computer, there are computers you can use at public libraries throughout the country. If you don't know how to use a computer, there are computer classes run by libraries and universities. Or you can hire a teenager or other computer geek to get you started. Never has so much information been available with such ease, at the press of your finger. So, enjoy!

You might even want to start your own Web site or blog. It is easy to do and inexpensive. You will never look back.

Don't Do Just One Thing, or Be Just One Person

Furthermore, you don't have to do just one thing, or be just one person. You can be a parent, a spouse, an expert, a consultant, a friend, a confidant, a writer, a golfer, a dreamer—please make your own list, and pursue those identities and activities that intrigue you. And you can add identities and activities as you get to know yourself better. (See Chapter 12 for additional interesting approaches to discovering hidden aspects of yourself.)

The fact is that you can be anything you want to be in your old age. You don't have to worry about being a failure at what you try to do, because there is no such thing as failure when you are retired. If you don't like what you're trying to do, or if you realize it really cannot be done, there are other choices open to you. It is simply a matter of finding what will satisfy you.

And then, of course, there is grandparenting. We could devote an entire chapter specifically to grandparenting. Grandparents and grandchildren are "each other's treasures." You can play with your grandchildren, spoil them, teach them, guide them, talk with them, exchange gifts with them, and many more things. You are now free to spend more time with them, wherever they live. You can visit them, start an e-mail correspondence, talk to them on the phone, or even talk with them via modern technologies, such as Skype. Many more forms of communication are continuously being invented.

I have mentioned only a few of the options available to you, but remember that you have an unlimited number of more options as never before in your life. Explore them; indulge in them. It is all out there for the asking, so ask!

Chapter Summary

- You are now in a new phase of your life.
- You will first of all want to be yourself.
- What are some of the building blocks for a changed identity?
- What are you going to do in retirement?
- You can keep doing what you have been doing.
- You can start to do something brand new.
- Learn a new skill.
- Teach what you know.
- Write your autobiography.
- Travel the world.
- Google the world.
- Don't do just one thing, or be just one person.

Chapter 5

Make Your Relationships and Social Life a High Priority

WE HUMANS are social animals. From day one we could not survive without someone to care for us, which is usually a mother. We do better with two caretakers, often a mother and a father. Growth and learning take place only in a social setting. We need social connections throughout life.

In this chapter we talk about many kinds of social relationships, but especially those that assume greatest significance in your later years. Early in life our social relationships with our parents matter most. Later in life the circle of social relationships enlarges, through school, work, as well as leisure activities, and, in most cases, then one relationship emerges as your most important one: that with your spouse or partner.

I am going to surmise that your spouse is now the most important person in your life. I assume this because: (1) you *chose* him or her; (2) you may have spent more time with that person than with any other person in your life; (3) in your later years, especially after one or both of you retire, you *will* spend even more time with your spouse or partner than with any other person; and (4) research has shown that having a spouse has tremendous survival value: married people far outlive those who are widowed, separated, or divorced. For that reason, and many more, it is very important to take good care of your spouse! It might even rank as one of the most important things to do in your retirement. Accordingly, now is the time to aim to perfect this, your most important social relationship.

Aim to Perfect Your Most Important Social Relationship

To *perfect* anything is a tall order, but it is worth the effort to perfect your relationship with your spouse or partner. If you come even close, it will make a difference in the overall life satisfaction for both of you. Talk to each other about how you want to spend these later years. Identify those areas where you have common goals, and acknowledge those areas in which you want to go in different directions. Both things are possible; after all, you are not identical twins. The time to do this is now, while each of you can make changes and adjustments. And both of you need to agree on one goal: to take care of one another, as though your life depended on it. It does. You will need to be there for each other, in sickness and in health. Now is when it will really matter. There are many areas in which you can do things better together: socialize together; exercise together; make lifestyle changes together; travel together; spend time with the grandchildren together.

And naturally there will be areas of your lives that you explore separately: in creative expression, in what you read, in learning different new skills, in volunteer activities, in starting or running a business, and many other areas that you will discover now that you have more free time on your hands. This will give you new things to talk about, as you share your separate experiences with each other.

Prepare to Cope with Losses

Along with losing one's work associates when you retire, you lose many of your work-related social connections. You may find that your circle of contacts shrinks significantly. You may lose other social connections as well; for instance, if you or your friends move after retiring. So you get the picture: losses are ubiquitous. But what I focus on here is not so much the fact that such losses occur, but *how to cope with losses.*

The way to cope with losses is to restore some of the losses, but not to seek to restore all of them. What does that mean? After you retire, you may choose to maintain ongoing social relationships with *some* of your colleagues, but certainly not all of them. *Some* of these contacts could be replaced by new relationships that may come from entirely new social circles. This may involve converting mere acquaintances into friends. You may begin to socialize with your children as parent-to-child relationships become adult-to-adult relationships. Casual relationships with neighbors may blossom into real friendships as well. For those who choose to live in a new community, it may involve starting entirely new relationships and finding commonalities or even differences between these new friends that one can enjoy. More about the need for a larger circle of social connections will be discussed later on in this chapter.

Losing Your Most Important Relationship

What happens if you lose your spouse or partner through death or divorce or the ending of the relationship? It leaves a big hole in your life. How do you cope with it? First, you need to thoroughly *grieve* the loss.

Grieving the loss of a life partner or spouse is normal, and it takes time, anywhere from a few months to a few years. Grieving involves recalling all the valued aspects of the lost relationship. For some people this process includes what has been called sanctification—attributing even more positive characteristics to the person than he or she actually possessed. Grieving may also mean coming to terms with some of the imperfections that occur in most relationships.

Normal grief involves feelings of sadness and emptiness occasioned by the loss. Weeping is common, and may be best if done in the presence of close friends or relatives rather than when alone. Real relief can come from crying in the presence of a confidant. Some people feel like crying but are unable to cry, an even more painful experience. Sometimes, when grief is not resolved, it can lead to depression (more about depression in Chapter 7). At some point the grieving process must wind down in order for you to move on with your life. This means resuming an active social life or re-engaging in your community in a new role without a partner.

For some people, moving on with one's life may mean starting to "date" again. I put "date" in quotes because starting a new relationship after having been in a long-term relationship for many years is very different from dating as one remembers it from youth. It is unnerving. It feels strange. Yet it can be very satisfying to begin a relationship with a new partner. Yes, there I said it—sex! Some people will even consider marrying again, while others will decide to live together.

Retirement Marriages

The idea of remarriage can be a daunting one but one worth contemplating: for sheer survival value, for companionship, for intimacy, for sex, for sharing the day-to-day responsibilities of a household, and as an escape from loneliness. Not that it is easy to get remarried, or even probable. Most people who become widowed or divorced in old age will never remarry. They will have to adapt to widowhood as best they can, and more about that later.

First of all, you will meet other people who themselves are widowed. You may meet them if you join a grief support group, or you may know them already as part of your current social circle. Second, another widowed person may have some of the same needs you have. They, too, may be seeking to reestablish an ongoing intimate relationship. I have observed many happy retirement marriages. Some of these couples have been inordinately pleased with their decision to remarry. One couple, who found one another living in the same retirement community, put it to me this way: "Our first marriage was the main meal; this is the dessert." Many other couples have shared similar expressions of satisfaction and delight.

A few bits of advice: If you have children and plan to remarry, discuss it with them. Discuss with them and with your future spouse how you plan to distribute your earthly goods after your death, whether it will be to your children, to your spouse, or some reasonable division between the two. Consider drafting and signing a prenuptial agreement that lays out these plans so that everything is clear to your children, to your new spouse, and to your new spouse's children. You could avoid future pain and disagreements between family members.

Living with a Significant Other

There is, perhaps increasingly so, yet another approach to replacing the loss of a spouse: living together with a new "significant other" without marrying. For a variety of reasons the new couple may not wish to marry. They may not want to disturb their current pattern of receiving a pension or Social Security income; or they may come from differing economic circumstances; or they may feel that a new legal arrangement is not necessary. As long as there is a strong commitment to one another, and both partners agree with this, living together can be a very satisfying solution for this part of your life. Of course, this, too, is very important to discuss with your children and also the children of your significant other.

Significant Other, Late in Life
We came together
Late in life
Two rivers mingling
Where each had been
Apart and unaware
Now flowing
As one
Our bond
Holier than holy
Impossible to rend
Bound for
A common sea

Going It Alone

Not everyone who becomes widowed or divorced or alone late in life is going to seek to remarry or to establish a new, committed relationship. By choice or by necessity, many older persons will spend their later years living alone, without the benefits or the burdens of a romantic relationship. If there is one word that characterizes the attitude of those who *choose* not to be involved in a new relationship, it is the word *freedom;* freedom from doing someone else's bidding; freedom from doing someone else's laundry; freedom to hold their own TV remote. Many unmarried older persons, especially some older women, *relish* this newfound freedom, and wouldn't give it up for anything. To some of them it is like a totally new revelation: they can do whatever they want, whenever they want, without asking permission from anyone. Of course, this may speak as much about some of the strictures of the relationship from which they were "liberated." I know of one woman who referred to those previously married and now living alone as "the new royalty," which simply reinforces the concept that people need to find what works *for them.*

More commonly, many men and a much larger number of women will spend their remaining years as widowers and widows. They will make peace with this status and establish other meaningful relationships that meet many if not all of their social needs. Some widows or widowers will go to live with their adult children or a sibling, or move into a retirement community where they can have as many social contacts on a daily basis as they wish.

Be Part of a Larger Social Network

Romantic relationships aside, participation in a larger social network is very important; in fact, it's necessary. Without that, you (or you and your partner) risk isolation, with all the negatives inherent therein. Having extensive social connections has survival value. Research studies have shown that individuals with extensive social connections tend to outlive those with fewer connections, and they tend to be happier and more contented. This view is universal. A proverb from Okinawa, a Japanese island with one of the longest-lived populations on the globe, states: "One cannot live in this world without the support of others."

As to the specifics of your social relationships, you can decide to which social networks you want to belong. For instance, you may wish to have many different levels of relationships with your extended family. One widow of my acquaintance is frequently in touch with all of her grandchildren, through mutual visiting, frequent phone calls, e-mails, or even such high-tech means as Skype or similar videophone contacts. You may belong to a church or synagogue, and participate in weekly services as well as committee meetings, lunches, working parties, volunteer activities, and so on. Or you may join, or start, a common interest group, such as a book club, a garden club, a card-playing group, a golfing partnership, or any of a dozen other possibilities. Just visiting regularly with your neighbor can be rewarding. By definition, neighbors are already close by; they are likely to share some common interests, but they are also likely to be of varied ages and interests, which can be very stimulating. Having this wider circle of social connections can mean that, along with my former patient, you too can say, "I am not alone."

Grandparents and Grandchildren Are Each Other's Treasures

Most people who have raised a child look forward to having grandchildren. If you are so blessed, establish special relationships with your grandchildren, regardless of where they live. Grandparents and grandchildren can truly be each other's treasures. Free of both parental and filial responsibilities, grandparents and grandchildren can forge their own special relationships, in person or by long distance. We live in a global village nowadays, and connecting with one another can be done by landline, by cell phone, by Skype, or by exchanging CDs or videotapes. As a grandparent, you may have more time for your grandchildren than their busy parents. Grandparents and grandchildren are often more accepting and less critical of each other than children and parents can be with each other. Often a child's first e-mail correspondence will be with a grandparent, and grandparents can shower both love and presents on their grandchildren, read to them, or introduce them to new activities. And it can work the other way around as well, to everyone's pleasure.

My wife maintains a special e-mail relationship with our granddaughter, Cassie. Though Cassie is 10 years old, she has a long ways to go toward being a good speller. She uses texting shortcuts, with no attention to grammar or spelling. In response to being asked to put more periods into her e-mails, Cassie responded (the grammar and spelling errors are all hers): "Well because I haven't been putting periods ill give you some . . . . there." A recent e-mail from Cassie was particularly amusing: "Grandma, please email to me im so mad im crying why do my parents have to be so mean." Half an hour later she wrote: "Forget what I wrote im going swimming with Jane."

Sometimes grandchildren invent unique and endearing names for their grandmother or grandfather.

Some of these names may start as mispronunciations, or they may be culturally determined variations on grandmother or grandfather, such as Abuela, Maw-Maw, Mutti, Nana, Opa, Pop-Pop, or still other intriguing variations that may bring both pleasure and an additional identity to the older person. If you haven't been in contact with your grandchildren lately, try it—you'll like it.

Pets Are Social Animals Too

For many people, young and old alike, pets are an integral part of their social relationships. Some people prefer cats as pets, while some people prefer dogs; some thrive on having both cats and dogs, while still others choose not to have pets at all. It is clearly a personal preference. But, as some social relationships drop out in the later years, pets can assume added significance.

> Boots is our Maine coon cat. He has been with us for six years. We have always had one or more cats in our household, as long as we have been married. But Boots is of special importance to us. He came to us when his former fam-

ily had to give him up when they relocated to
Hawaii and were unable to take him with them.

Boots is simply a love. He is sleek, fluffy, and
handsome, with an enormous tail. Throughout
the day he stays close to one or both of us
and lies languorously on chairs and tables by
the hour. It is simply impossible to pass him
without petting or cuddling him. At night, he
sleeps between us at the head of our bed, turn-
ing sometimes to one, then to the other, for
attention. He awakens one or another of us to
let him out into the yard toward morning, and
then waits eagerly to be let in when we arise.
We could not imagine being without him,
although he is now more than ten years old.
We both know that he will be with us for only
a few more years. When he leaves us, we hope
we can find another cat as nearly like him as
possible.

There you have it: Social relationships are very important for your happiness, your health, your survival, and
just for fun. Social relationships don't cost very much in
terms of dollars and cents, but they pay terrific dividends
in smiles, personal satisfaction, and well-being.

Chapter Summary

- We are all social animals.
- Perfect your most important social relationship.
- Retirement marriages can be as satisfying as any other marriage.
- Consider living with a "significant other."
- Going it alone can offer newfound freedom.
- Be part of a larger social network.
- Grandchildren and grandparents are each other's treasures.
- Your pets are social animals too.

Chapter 6

Insist on Good Health—
Everything Else Depends On It

GOOD HEALTH is a prerequisite for successful aging. It is necessary for everything you will want to do in retirement. Accordingly, maintaining and even improving your health status in your later years is a high priority. Good health has been described as the ultimate aphrodisiac.

Even if you have been healthy all of your life, do not take your good health for granted. You cannot expect to stay healthy and free of all illness as you age. You may be faced with an acute or chronic illness at any time, and your responsibility will be to deal with it aggressively. Acute illnesses need to be *treated* completely; chronic illnesses need to be *managed* aggressively so as to minimize limitations and functional impairment.

You need to be very much in charge of your own health care, learning to understand and to manage any illnesses and conditions that arise. So, where do you start?

This chapter is divided into two parts: the first covers issues related to health care in general and the second covers issues related to specific diseases or conditions. The first portion definitely applies to everyone, as it discusses attitudes and approaches to health care in general, but the discussion of specific illnesses and conditions may or may not apply. Since it is likely that you will experience one or more of these illnesses during your later years, this section may be worth a quick skim so that you know which issues are covered. You can then return to those sections as they apply specifically to you. So here's to your health!

Issues Related to Your Health Care in General

Establish a Strong Relationship with a Well-Qualified Primary Care Physician

First, you must find a skilled and experienced *primary care doctor* with whom you can communicate easily, and who shares with you the philosophy that acute illnesses are to be treated vigorously and chronic illnesses are to be managed aggressively. Your primary care physician can be someone trained in family medicine, internal medicine, or one of the internal medical specialties. He or she will take responsibility for an initial evaluation and periodic visits and will also handle coordination and referrals to any specialty physicians. Any specialty physician in turn will keep your primary care physician informed of all diagnostic or treatment procedures carried out by the specialist.

Obtain the Best Health Insurance Coverage You Can Afford

In order to receive great health care, you have to have great health care insurance. You cannot afford *not* to have good health insurance coverage. A lack of such coverage could break you physically and financially, as I illustrate throughout this chapter.

You Must Have Medicare

Medicare will cover most individuals over age 65 for both hospital services (Medicare Part A) and outpatient medical services (Medicare Part B). But Medicare alone is not enough. In addition you must—and this is an absolute must—have strong secondary or supplemental health insurance to cover all or most of the costs that are not covered by Medicare. Such secondary or supplemental insurance must be with a reputable, well-established corporation, such as Blue Cross/Blue Shield or another trustworthy, national company, such as those available through AARP (American Association of Retired Persons).

It is also important that you fully understand the importance of receiving your health care *within the network* covered by your primary and secondary insurance carrier. Costs of "out-of-network" medical care can be prohibitive. The following story illustrates the importance of having both Medicare and a Medicare supplement policy:

> Helen, age 70, experienced a few extra heartbeats that caused her concern. She went to see her primary care doctor, who reassured her that it was "probably nothing to worry about" but nevertheless recommended that Helen have a cardiac stress test. She was referred to the diagnostic center of a local hospital and the test was performed. It took more than four hours, and at the end of it the technician expressed the opinion that "everything was normal" and

her primary care doctor confirmed that the test was "negative."

Helen was surprised when, two weeks later, she received a statement from the hospital billing department listing the test she had had at a cost of $7,900, and there might be additional charges for the professional services of a cardiologist. In very fine print, which she did not read the first time she looked at the bill, it did say that she didn't need to do anything about the bill until the hospital had heard from her insurance company, and that then she would be responsible for whatever "residual charges" were left. Eventually she learned that while the charges for the test had been $7,900, the Medicare "allowable" amount was only $1,795.50, and that Medicare eventually paid 80 percent of this amount to the hospital, and her secondary insurance company, in her case Blue Cross/Blue Shield, had paid the remaining 20 percent of the allowable charges. The final amount of "out-of-pocket" charges owed by Helen was $0.00. What a relief!

Now imagine, however, that Helen did not have Medicare and a secondary health insurance policy. The hospital would seek to recover the full amount of their charges ($7,900) from Helen, which would far exceed her resources. This difference between "charges" made by a health care provider and the amount "allowed" by Medicare or another insurance company is one of the things that is very much wrong with the current health care system. It remains to be seen to what extent this problem will be addressed or even remedied by the current spate of health care reform efforts being made by the federal government. But for now, however, this story clearly shows how uncovered medical expenses can be a real danger to the financial status of any elderly person.

Read Explanation of Benefits Statements (EOBs) from Medicare and Other Insurance Companies with Great Care, and If Need Be, Challenge These Statements

In dealing with Medicare and other health insurance companies, it is vitally important that you fully understand Explanation of Benefits statements (EOBs) and, if need be, challenge them. Although all such statements have presumably been coordinated, they often are not, and you may be told that you need to pay monies that have already been or will be paid by the insurance companies. You need to have a clear understanding of which insurance company is your primary insurance company and which is secondary. In general, your primary insurance company should be billed first, and the remainder of the bill sent to the secondary insurance company. However, this does not always happen in the proper order. If you feel that a claim has been improperly denied, each insurance company has its own unique appeals process that you can use to have a claim reconsidered for payment. Since medical care can make up quite a high proportion of your expenses, you must be fully informed and nimble in dealing with these organizations so that you won't be overcharged.

Know All the Facts Before You Join a Health Maintenance Organization (HMO)

Health Maintenance Organizations provide health care based on Medicare benefits plus other promised services, such as preventive services. The advantages of HMOs in general are their low cost and the fact that they promise to cover all your acute (but not long-term) health care needs, including the cost of medications. The disadvantages are that the HMO, not you, and not your doctor, determines what services you will receive and what doctors you may consult, and when you may consult a specialist. HMOs are operated for profit, and financial considerations benefiting the HMO are sometimes—though not always—the overriding determiners of the kind of care you will receive. Again, explore and compare—and beware! It is your health that is on the line. Few decisions are more important than the kind of health care coverage you and your family have in old age.

Deal Aggressively and Completely with Acute Illnesses

Your approach to any acute illness has to be vigorous and complete. Possible acute illnesses include colds, flu, upper respiratory infections, sinusitis, pneumonia, urinary tract infection, heart attacks, strokes and transient ischemic attacks (TIAs), and a flock of others that I will discuss. Your primary care doctor needs to know about and advise on or treat any of these conditions. Your care may eventually involve medical specialists, such as a cardiologist, endocrinologist, neurologist, or urologist. However, such care by a medical specialist should be initiated by your primary care doctor. Once a relationship with a medical specialist has been established, you may continue to receive care directly from that specialist. You should request, however, that the specialist keep your primary care doctor informed of whatever diagnostic or treatment procedures are implemented.

Deal Aggressively and Completely with Chronic Illnesses

Examples of chronic illnesses include diabetes, hypertension, coronary artery disease, congestive heart failure, arthritis, and osteoporosis, to mention only a few that I discuss in some detail in this chapter. Some less common illnesses are dealt with in the Appendix (pages 249–293). For each and every one of the chronic illnesses that you may develop, it will behoove you to fully understand that illness in detail, including treatment options, complications, etc. So you may want to search the Internet or buy a book on that specific illness, as recommended by your primary care physician.

How to Deal with Accidents or Injuries

Obviously, it would be best to avoid accidents and injuries, so avoid high-risk behaviors, such as "showing off" or participating in sports with a high risk of injuries, and make a point of driving so as to avoid accidents and fall-proofing your home so as to avoid injuries from falls. But even when precautions are taken, accidents or injuries may still nevertheless occur. Accidents and significant injuries are most appropriately treated in a hospital emergency room. Minor injuries, though, can probably be treated by your primary care doctor.

Insist on Complete Healing and Recovery after Illnesses or Injuries

Dr. Julie Silver, a rehabilitation specialist at Harvard Medical School and a breast cancer survivor, has written an entire book on the topic of healing completely, titled *Super Healing*. Silver makes the point that *complete* recovery is the ultimate goal following the treatment for any injury or illness, and that it often requires some additional special efforts. She cites four elements essential to bringing about complete recovery or super healing:

1. Regular meals, specifically five small meals a day, each with sufficient protein and fruits and vegetables.

2. Stress reduction, using meditation, muscle relaxation, yoga, or prayer.
3. Loving relationships.
4. Physical activity to rebuild muscles, strength, and self-confidence. To effect full recovery from a major accident or illness such as a stroke, a period of rehabilitation may need to follow the acute treatment of the disease or accident.

Avoid Unnecessary Hospitalizations

Certain illnesses and conditions can be treated only in hospitals. Among these are heart attacks, strokes, severe infectious diseases, and anything that requires major surgery. However, you should do everything in your power to avoid unnecessary hospitalizations for these reasons:

1. Hospitalizations are expensive.
2. Hospitalizations expose you to risk of hospital-borne infections and hospital-based medical errors.
3. Hospitalization involves inactivity, which robs you of muscle mass, which might then require follow-up rehab care. Instead, work closely with your primary care physician to

use preventive and early-intervention approaches that minimize hospitalizations.

Make Lifestyle Choices That Reduce the Risk of Common Chronic Diseases

Research shows that there are relatively simple lifestyle choices you can make to reduce the risk of some of the most common chronic diseases, such as diabetes, heart disease, and high blood pressure. You might think of these choices as the *Ten Commandments of Wellness.*

THE TEN COMMANDMENTS OF WELLNESS

1. Engage in vigorous exercise every day of your life.
2. Eat a heart-healthy diet.
3. Avoid becoming overweight.
4. Do not smoke.
5. Use alcohol only in moderation.
6. Get seven to eight hours of sleep every night.
7. Develop a mechanism for stress reduction that works for you.
8. Remain socially active and involved.
9. Reduce risk-taking behaviors.
10. Get vaccinated against the flu every year and

against shingles and pneumococcal pneumonia once in your later years.

You can add bonus commandments to this list to re-
flect your unique individuality by doing whatever else
you believe will keep you healthy.

Now let us discuss each of these "commandments"
in detail:

1. *Engage in vigorous exercise every day of your life.* This
topic will be dealt with in a separate chapter, Chapter 10.

2. *Eat a heart-healthy diet.* A great deal has been written
about an ideal diet, much of it confusing and contradictory. My advice: Eat a Mediterranean-style diet. This diet
contains large amounts of fruits and vegetables, whole
grains, beans, nuts, fish, relatively little red meat, and
uses olive oil as the most important source of fat. If you
like, add a glass of red wine to your evening meal. Calories should be limited to 1,800 calories for women and
2,000 calories for men, to either maintain or slightly
reduce weight. What to do if you are overweight?

3. *Avoid becoming overweight.* You cannot afford to become or to remain overweight. Observing the first and
the second "commandments" (exercise and a heart-
healthy diet) will keep you from becoming overweight,

or, if you are overweight, commit to habitual daily exercise and a heart-healthy diet, with calories not to exceed 1,800 calories per day, which will allow you to gradually reduce your weight. But being overweight alone is not the problem; you need to reduce the proportion of your body weight that is fat and increase the proportion of muscle. Being overweight is serious business indeed, as it increases the risks of many illnesses, limits your mobility, and makes you look and feel less attractive than you could be.

4. *Don't smoke.* This recommendation has been around for a very long time, yet it still needs to be restated for those relatively few people who still smoke in their later years. It is never too late to benefit from quitting smoking altogether. I am talking here about complete cessation of smoking, not merely cutting down. The research data for this is overwhelming, and relatively effective smoking-cessation techniques are now available. Remember that a journey of a thousand miles starts with a decision:

Leslie is a 67-year-old woman who, despite everything she knows about the dangers of smoking, still smokes. Her skin is prematurely old. She speaks with a gravelly voice, and she becomes short of breath when she exerts herself. Her smoking is a constant irritation to her husband, who never smoked, and her smoking triggers many arguments between them. In addition, her smoking makes her a poor role model for her children and grandchildren, and she exposes them regularly to the risks of secondary smoke. As a friend of the family, I have tried to persuade her to undergo a smoking-cessation program, but thus far have not been successful. But I will keep on trying.

5. *Use alcohol only in moderation.* The use of alcohol in the later years has also been subject to a lot of conflicting information. Again, the best advice I can give you is to continue to abstain from alcohol if you have never used alcohol until now. On the other hand, if you have been accustomed to drinking socially, say, two martinis with dinner, my best advice to you is that it is time to change: have no more than one drink no more than several times a week. Having two martinis in your 60s, 70s, or 80s is like having four martinis when you were younger. Of course, there are a lot of positive things to be said about using alcohol *in moderation:* it helps socialization, it relaxes you, and the poets have sung the ben-

efits of drink for a long time. One of my favorite poets, Li Po, wrote: "Such is the rapture of wine, that the sober shall never inherit."

6. *Get seven to eight hours of sleep every night.* Sleep is the great restorer. You absolutely need seven to eight hours of sleep a day or your body will not be able to catch up with you. How can you assure good sleep? Practice good sleep hygiene! This means physical activity during the day; no caffeine after 1:00 PM; winding down your day's activities and worries several hours before sleep; going to bed at the same time every night; doing nothing in your bedroom except sleep (sex excepted). Alcohol as a sleep inducer does not work, as it makes you sleepy at bedtime, only to arouse you a few hours later.

7. *Develop a method for stress reduction that works for you.* There are many ways to practice stress reduction, and you need to determine which methods work best for you. These may include relaxation exercises, listening to soothing music, meditation, various forms of yoga, or whatever you have learned that allows you to clear the conflicts of the day out of your brain and allow the great restorer to take over. A word about sleeping medications: If you need to use them, use them occasionally only. They lose their effect if used regularly. They can be

addicting, in that you need larger and larger doses, as your body becomes tolerant to the medications.

8. *Remain socially active and involved.* I've already covered the need to remain socially active in Chapter 5.

9. *Reduce risk-taking behaviors.* Your later years are not for taking chances. You need to know the limits of your capabilities and not exceed them. Taking someone up on a dare or showing off puts you at a dangerous and unnecessary risk. If you want to expand your capabilities, you need to go into training. Bones are more fragile. Balance is less secure. Vision and hearing impairments may contribute to your vulnerabilities. Know yourself!

10. *Get vaccinated.* Be sure to get vaccinated against the flu every year, and against shingles and pneumococcal pneumonia once in your later years. Keep your tetanus vaccine up to date (once every ten years).

YOUR BONUS COMMANDMENTS OF WELLNESS

Well, here you are on your own. You may have discovered some special secrets, or your mother may have given you some very good advice about what to do or what not to do. Share it with me by e-mail at epfeiffe@ health.usf.edu so I can continue to learn what works and what doesn't. I would appreciate it, and maybe in the next edition, your commandment will replace or be added to those that now make up the Ten Commandments of Wellness. There is nothing magic about having 10 rules concerning wellness; it just allows us to invoke the authority of the Bible.

Be Your Own Health Care Manager

Nobody is as interested in or as committed to your good health as you are. Nobody benefits as much from maintaining your wellness as you do. For that reason, you need to become your own health care manager. Nobody can do it for you. This is a serious task, and it will require your attention every day.

Choose a Co-Manager of Your Health Care

To further indicate the importance of this issue, I have one other recommendation: *make your spouse, significant other, or a close friend the co-manager of your health care.* This becomes particularly valuable and necessary when you go to see your doctor. Your co-manager needs to know what issues are discussed and can be another set of ears and eyes to absorb important information.

The role of co-manager of your health care becomes even more urgent and necessary if you are ever hospitalized or go through any other type of complex procedure or treatment, like heart surgery or chemotherapy, which may make you less capable of supervising your own health care.

Know Your Numbers

One aspect of your task as your own health care manager is to "know your numbers." These are your vital statistics that you need to know and understand, and you need to take action if those numbers need improvements. The most important are blood pressure, heart rate, cholesterol levels, fasting blood sugar levels, weight and body mass index, and pedometer score.

BLOOD PRESSURE

Your blood pressure score is made up of two numbers, your systolic (higher) and your diastolic (lower) number. Both are important. Both high and low blood pressure can be dangerous to your health. Abnormally high blood pressure is associated with the risk of heart attack and stroke; abnormally low blood pressure is associated with the risk of fainting or falls. Normal blood pressure is considered to be 120 over 80, with a range of 105 to 120 for the systolic pressure and a range of 60 to 80 for the diastolic pressure. Blood pressures above or below these values are cause for serious concern and should be brought to your primary care doctor's attention for treatment.

HEART RATE

A normal heart rate at rest is between 60 and 80 beats per minute. Learn to determine your own heart rate. You do this by placing your index and middle finger of one hand over the wrist of the other hand, palm up, until you find the pulse. You can do this most easily by finding the small groove at the outside part of your wrist. Then count the number of beats over one minute. Unless you are an athlete in regular training, heart rates below 60 and heart rates above 80 beats per minute at rest should be a matter of concern for you and your doctor. By taking your own pulse rate, you will also be able to pick up any heart rhythm irregularity, such as multiple skipped beats, irregular heart rates, or extremely rapid heart rates. Again, these should be a matter of concern for you and your doctor. Of course, after activity your heart rates will be much higher, depending on the intensity of your activity.

CHOLESTEROL

Your cholesterol level, as determined by laboratory blood tests, should be below 200 mg/ml. Higher levels than that increase your risk of heart disease and hypertension significantly. Marked elevation of your cholesterol level, such as values over 250 or even over 300, should alarm you and your doctor, and you will need to begin a program for lowering your cholesterol level. This may include changes in diet, exercise level, and possibly the use of one or more medications for lowering cholesterol levels.

FASTING BLOOD SUGAR LEVELS

Fasting blood sugar levels should be between 80 and 110 mg. Levels higher or even much higher than that indicate the presence either of metabolic syndrome or diabetes. If you have diabetes, you must try to control your blood sugar levels to keep them within this range to avoid complications.

WEIGHT AND BODY MASS INDEX

Your weight should be maintained at the ideal weight calculated for your gender and your height. In addition, another measure, called the body mass index (BMI), should be maintained in the 20 to 25 range. The body mass index is calculated by taking your weight in pounds, dividing it by your height in inches squared, and multiplying this number by 703. Don't try to do this in your head—use a calculator. For instance, if you are 5 foot 10, or 70 inches tall, and your weight is 170 pounds, your body mass index would be calculated as follows: 170 divided by 70 squared, multiplied by 703. The result would be 170 divided by 4900 and multiplied by 703 = 24.39. BMI figures below 20 indicate that you're underweight, between 20 and 25 are normal or ideal, between 25 and 30 indicate overweight, and a number above 30 indicates outright obesity. For the mathematically challenged internet help is available to calculate your BMI, e.g. http://www.nhlbisupport.com/bmi.

PEDOMETER SCORE

You should get a pedometer to measure how many steps you take each day. Measuring steps should become part of your exercise regimen; keep track of the steps you take going about your regular daily activities, whether you're shopping, gardening, or visiting friends. Aim to walk at least 5,000 to 10,000 steps per day; anything beyond 10,000 steps is even better.

Additional Special Health Care Topics

Here are a few more bits of advice to make sure that you understand your own health situation: Make a list of questions that you want to ask your doctor and take notes on the doctor's answers. Ask questions of your doctors about anything that you don't understand. In addition, ask why diagnostic tests and procedures are necessary, and what they will accomplish.

There are two reasons for this advice. Many doctors are concerned about being sued for malpractice, and accordingly, may order an abundance of tests to make sure that they cannot be accused of neglect. That practice not only drives up your cost but also the cost of medical care nationally. Second, there is a huge discrepancy in how doctors are paid. Doctors who primarily practice what may be called "cognitive medicine," family practitioners, general internists, psychiatrists, and pediatricians, are paid for their knowledge and for their time. Doctors who make a livelihood by providing various "procedures" earn much higher incomes, as they are paid per procedure. The more procedures they perform, the better their bank account looks. Make sure you understand why a procedure, such as a colonoscopy, an MRI, or even a hospitalization, is necessary, so as not to contribute to the national burden and your personal burden of health care costs.

CONCIERGE MEDICINE

Concierge medicine is a new type of medical care that harkens back to a time when doctors could and did spend more time with their patients, and when patients could get an appointment whenever they needed it. In today's practice of medicine, doctor's appointments are frequently limited to no more than 15 minutes, and there can be long waits before the patient is actually seen. This has led to an excessive use of emergency room visits by people who feel they need immediate attention, and, again, a higher cost of medical care, both to the individual and to the national system. What concierge medicine seeks to provide is unlimited time for a thorough annual evaluation, a plan for preventive measures, same-day or next-day appointments, access to the doctor's cell phone number, and many other benefits. For these privileges, individuals may pay an annual fee, anywhere between $1,000 and $2,000 per year, and the doctor in turn agrees to take on no more than a limited number of patients, say 500 or 600 patients, compared to the usual case load of several thousands of patients. Enrolled patients are entitled to house calls when needed, a two-hour annual physical exam, and nutritional and fitness analysis and advice. It may include a "presidential physical" that mimics the kind of examination presidents of the United States receive.

Concierge or VIP medical care, as it is sometimes called, is not a substitute for health insurance coverage, as other aspects of medical care, such as setting a broken arm, hospitalization for a heart attack or stroke, or an elective procedure, will still need to be covered by regular medical insurance. However, the idea behind concierge medical care is that by emphasizing preventive care and easy access to a physician, problems such as diabetes, hypertension, stroke, or other situations requiring hospitalization may be minimized. (There is even a fictional TV program about concierge medicine called *Royal Pains* on the USA network.)

THE ELECTRONIC MEDICAL RECORD

Another issue that you may hear about increasingly is the electronic medical record (EMR). This is a technique in which all relevant medical information is contained in an electronic database that patients can carry with them and can easily be shared between treating physicians, hospitals, and other health care providers. Issues of compatibility between EMR systems and issues of confidentiality remain to be worked out in the next few years.

ESTABLISHMENT OF A HEALTH CARE ADVOCACY CORPS

Here I am suggesting a new volunteer service that will be of particular value as the nation begins to implement the health care reform package passed in the 2009 Congress: Volunteer community health care advocates. This would be a role for retired physicians, nurses, social workers, physical and occupational therapists, all of whom know and understand the health care system particularly well. They would be available to patients who are having difficulty navigating the new or the old health care network and would intervene as "friend-of-the-court" activists to get people the health care they need with a minimum of red tape and confusion.

Issues Related to Specific Diseases or Conditions

The following is an overview of diseases and conditions that are common among seniors and that you or your partner may cross paths with in the years ahead. This is by no means a complete medical description of any of these; anyone who suspects they may be affected by any of these conditions should see their doctor for a thorough evaluation.

Upper Respiratory Infections

Upper respiratory infections can include sinusitis, bronchitis, and pneumonia, depending on whether the sinuses, the bronchi, or the peripheral lung tissue is affected. Infections can be either bacterial or viral. Antibiotics are used in the treatment of bacterial infections. The offending agents in viral infections are less subject to eradication and are primarily dealt with through supportive measures, such as rest, plenty of fluid intake, anti-fever medication, and anti-inflammatory agents.

Urinary Tract Infections

Urinary tract infections are characterized by frequent urination, possibly accompanied by a burning sensation, flank pain, or pain in the lower abdomen, and sometimes by fever. Your primary care physician will confirm the diagnosis with a urinalysis, which will also provide information about the sensitivity of the infecting organism to specific antibiotics. Treatment consists of a course of appropriate antibiotics, based on a sensitivity test, and increased fluid intake to "wash out" the offending infection. A single episode should be followed by an investigation by your doctor into the cause of the infection, which could originate either in your bladder or your kidneys. This is particularly warranted if there are recurrent urinary tract infections.

Influenza (or Flu)

I have already recommended that you get a flu shot every fall from your doctor or a local pharmacy to minimize the likelihood of developing a case of influenza. In addition, it is important to pay attention to personal hygiene, such as washing your hands frequently, especially during the flu season. Influenza is generally characterized by fever, malaise, muscle aches and pains, respiratory symptoms such as a runny nose and sneezing, but there can frequently also be gastrointestinal symptoms such as nausea, vomiting, and diarrhea. Flu symptoms should be managed with bed rest, anti-fever medications such as acetaminophen (Tylenol), and ample fluid intake. Unless a specific bacterial "super infection" occurs, antibiotics are not useful in treating the flu. Avoid close contact with household members while infected to help prevent the spread of the disease. In certain years, specific strains of influenza can become epidemic, such as the "swine flu" in 2009 or the Asian (Hong Kong) flu in previous years. New, specific vaccines are usually developed in the case of such epidemics, and you should take this in addition to your regular seasonal flu shot.

Diabetes and Metabolic Syndrome (Pre-Diabetes)

Diabetes (and its precursor, metabolic syndrome) is one of the most significant chronic illnesses. I am talking here about Type II, or late-onset diabetes, not the Type I diabetes that starts in young individuals. Diabetes is a chronic metabolic disorder experienced by 15 to 20 percent of people over age 65. Risk factors contributing to the onset of diabetes are advancing age, caloric over-nutrition, and a sedentary lifestyle. Of course the predisposition for diabetes can also be inherited, as diabetes tends to run in families. Diabetes is a disorder in which the body is unable to metabolize glucose in an optimal way, leading to multiple symptoms and potential complications. Symptoms of diabetes include weight gain, excessive thirst, excessive urination, and fatigue. Complications of diabetes may include hypertension, coronary heart disease, kidney failure, diabetic neuropathy, and vision problems, as well as erectile deficiency in males. As with many of the chronic illnesses common in old age, diabetes may be treated with medications *and* lifestyle modifications. Lifestyle modifications include maintaining an ideal weight; getting regular vigorous exercise; avoiding refined carbohydrates (sugar, candies, and most other sugary desserts, white bread, and pasta); and replacing these with whole-grain carbohydrates, vegetables, nuts, and legumes.

Diabetes medications come in several categories, depending on the specific metabolic effects they produce. Included are drugs like Glucophage (generic is metformin), which help your body to better use glucose, drugs that lower insulin resistance (like Actos), and a few newer drugs that have a variety of effects. The goal of treatment is to maintain normal blood sugar levels and to avoid complications of diabetes.

Hypertension

Hypertension, or high blood pressure, is another common chronic condition affecting individuals as they age. Because it produces no symptoms, it is sometimes referred to as a silent killer. Untreated, it can give rise to multiple complications, the most serious of which are stroke, multiple transient ischemic attacks (TIAs), coronary artery disease, congestive heart failure, and kidney failure. Blood pressure is easily measured in the doctor's office or in one's own home. Anyone with a problem with high blood pressure should probably keep a reliable blood pressure monitor at home for frequent— if not daily—testing. It used to be said that older persons could be allowed mild elevations of systolic blood pressure, such increases being considered "normal." But as with many aspects of aging, "normal" is no longer good enough; the current view is that any significant elevation of blood pressure should be treated. Thus, systolic blood pressure (the higher of the two blood pressure numbers) should be maintained in the range between 105 and 120; diastolic pressure (the lower blood pressure number) should not exceed 80 and not drop below 60.

As is true with a number of the chronic illnesses, treatment of hypertension is approached through a combination of lifestyle changes *and* medications. Lifestyle changes include instigating a regular exercise program, a heart-healthy diet, losing excess body weight, and using stress-reduction techniques. If diet and exercise alone are not sufficient to control blood pressure, then one or more medications should be added to the treatment program.

The first type of medication usually tried is a diuretic, which helps the body rid itself of extra, retained water. If that alone is not sufficient, your doctor may put you on medications with additional mechanisms of action to bring about effective blood pressure control. This needs to be done gradually to avoid sudden drops in blood pressure, or drops in blood pressure when arising, so-called orthostatic hypertension. These sudden drops can be dangerous, as they may lead to fainting or falls, both of which can lead to injury.

Other types of medication your doctor may place you on for high blood pressure include beta-blockers, ACE inhibitors, or anti-rennin medications. Your doctor will advise you on which type of medication you need and how to take these medications. Since all medications have potential side effects, it is desirable to accomplish lowering your blood pressure through lifestyle modifications, minimizing the use of medications. If you do need to take medications, take them exactly as prescribed by your doctor.

Coronary Artery Disease

Coronary artery disease or coronary heart disease is defined as obstruction of the coronary arteries, which are the arteries that supply blood to the heart muscle itself. Two types of manifestations are most prominent. The first of these is angina pectoris, or angina, for brief. This is pain in the chest, often radiating down to the left arm, upon exertion. The other is myocardial infarction, or a heart attack, when one or another of the coronary arteries is blocked, and the heart muscle area supplied by that artery suffers damage. Again, a number of lifestyle changes may be recommended to deal with these risks, including a heart-healthy diet, moderate but regular exercise, and weight control. A variety of medications are available to reduce the symptoms of angina, such as nitroglycerin tablets. A heart attack requires immediate hospitalization and a period of rest to allow healing, followed by a resumption of activities to regain both heart and muscle strength.

Another group of heart problems that may be age-related or related to coronary artery disease are irregular heart rhythms, such as atrial fibrillation, other irregular heartbeats, or excessively rapid heart rates. This condition too needs to be treated, as untreated arrhythmias may increase the risk of heart attacks and stroke.

Congestive Heart Failure

Congestive heart failure is caused when the heart muscle starts to weaken. This may be due to systemic hypertension, pulmonary hypertension, or coronary artery disease, with one or more cardiac infarctions. The principal symptoms of congestive heart failure are shortness of breath on exertion and inability to lie flat in bed as excessive fluid accumulates in the lungs. A number of medications are available to strengthen heart muscle action, the most prominent among these being digitalis preparations. But diuretics, which remove excess fluid from the blood stream, may also be useful to reduce symptoms. Since congestive heart failure severely limits exercise tolerance, it too must be treated vigorously when it occurs. Again, the best treatment would be prevention, and here the various lifestyle measures, which have already been discussed, will work to minimize the risk of heart failure.

Strokes and Transient Ischemic Attacks (TIA)

A stroke is the result of a blockage of an artery supplying one or more areas of the brain. A stroke results in loss of function of muscles, speech, or sensation in one part of the body depending on what portion of the brain is affected. A stroke has also been called a "brain attack," in analogy to a heart attack, to emphasize the critical nature of the event and the need for rapid intervention. If you suspect that you are having a stroke, you must get to an emergency room immediately. There doctors will evaluate the nature of the stroke and determine whether administering a clot-dissolving medication can reverse the arterial blockage. If the clot can't be dissolved in a timely manner, the portion of the brain to which the blood supply is blocked will die. Rehabilitation can often help recover lost function through the transfer of functions from the infarcted area to another part of the brain.

Chronic Pulmonary Disease

The principal chronic pulmonary disease is emphysema, also called chronic obstructive pulmonary disease, or COPD for short. In COPD, shortness of breath is caused by constriction of the bronchi, which reduces the amount of air entering the lungs. Emphysema may be caused by smoking, by chronic dust inhalation, or by exposure to other hazardous gases. Since COPD limits function, vigorous treatment must be pursued. This may include the use of inhalers to open up the airflow to the lungs. Vigorous treatment of both acute and chronic infections of the lungs is also indicated when it occurs.

Cancer

Cancer, of course, is one of the most feared illnesses. Cancer is an abnormal tissue growth that, unless controlled or removed surgically, will threaten adjoining tissues and may lead to death. Eternal vigilance to any abnormal growth is necessary on both the part of the patient and the doctor. Cancer must be detected and removed as early as possible, before it has a chance to spread or metastasize to other parts of the body. The most common cancers are cancer of the lung, the colon, and the breast in women and of the prostate in men.

The most effective treatment of cancers is excision of the offending tumor. When this cannot be done in time, both radiation and chemotherapy can play an important role in slowing or stopping the growth of cancerous tissue. Because radiation and chemotherapy can cause "collateral damage" to cells other than cancer cells, both must be carefully "targeted" in order to limit damage to other tissues. Radiation and chemotherapy primarily affect growing or dividing cells. Thus, collateral damage may include damage to bone marrow, cells in the gastro-intestinal tract, and hair growth. Cancer care is, for the most part, the domain of cancer specialists, or oncologists, but your primary care doctor has a critical role to play in supervising the treatment strategies involved. And, as always, you yourself will need to be your own principal health care manager. So, if you are affected by cancer, you need to become thoroughly knowledgeable on the specific form of cancer affecting you. That way you will be able to maximally assist your doctors in your treatment.

Arthritis

Chronic arthritis is inflammation, stiffening, and calcification of the body's joints. Symptoms include limited range of motion and pain. The most common form of arthritis is chronic osteoarthritis. This can affect any of the joints of the body: joints in the hands, feet, hips, and spine. Today, no effective means of prevention or cure are available. Treatment consists primarily of controlling pain, lessening of inflammation, and mildly exercising the affected joints. More and more, joint-replacement strategies, such as hip joint, knee joint, and increasingly shoulder joint replacement, should be considered when symptomatic treatments alone are insufficient. These "parts replacement" strategies are becoming progressively simpler, more elegant, and less fraught with complications than in the past. Short of replacement therapies, anti-inflammatory medications are the principal treatment of arthritis. All of these medications carry a risk, as they can cause excessive bleeding of both the intestines and the skin. Non-anti-inflammatory pain medications, such as acetaminophen (Tylenol), can play an important role in pain control. Much touted, but still of limited proven usefulness, are glucosamine and chondroitin pills.

Obviously, I have covered only the most common acute and chronic illnesses. Less common acute and chronic illnesses are addressed in the Appendix. You may, of course, experience none or one or two of these illnesses. My recommendation is that you become an expert on whatever disease or condition from which you suffer, and that you work closely with your health care providers to manage them.

Chapter Summary

- **Insist on maintaining your health; everything else depends on it.**
- **Establish a strong relationship with a well-qualified primary care physician.**

- Obtain the best health insurance coverage you can afford.
- You must have Medicare.
- Medicare alone is not enough.
- Know all the facts before you join a health maintenance organization (HMO).
- Deal aggressively and completely with acute illnesses.
- Deal aggressively and completely with chronic illnesses.
- Know how to deal with accidents and injuries.
- Insist on complete healing and recovery from any accident or illness.
- Make these lifestyle changes: obey the ten commandments of wellness.
- Become your own health care manager.
- Make your spouse, significant other, or a close friend your health care co-manager.
- Know and understand every medicine you are taking: what it is for, what are the side effects, and how it may interact with other medicines you are taking.
- Understand the most common acute illnesses.
- Understand the most common chronic illnesses.

Chapter 7

Stay Mentally Healthy

AT THE OPENING session of the 2008 Annual Meeting of the American Psychiatric Association in San Francisco, the association's president asserted: "There is no health without mental health." I certainly agree with that statement. Accordingly, this chapter focuses on the important topic of mental health. It covers three aspects of mental health: (1) positive, or optimal, mental health; (2) mental health problems that can arise in later life; and (3) unique features related to the treatment of mental health problems. Let us first talk about positive mental health.

Positive Mental Health

Positive, or optimal, mental health can be defined as the zest that gives meaning and enjoyment to every act and every activity that we undertake. It needs to be nourished and guarded carefully. There are many aspects to positive mental health: self-esteem, a positive mood, an adequate level of energy, good memory and decision-making capacity, flexibility to adapt to whatever happens, and resiliency to bounce back from whatever adversity befalls us. A generally happy disposition is yet another aspect of positive mental health.

In a sense, mental health is a very fragile aspect of one's personality that can be fairly easily derailed through illness, personal losses, insufficient opportunity, or limited mobility. Chapter 16 discusses how "everything is related to everything else." Positive mental health is related to good physical health, good social connections, adequate income, suitable housing, good community amenities, and good spiritual support. It is probably acquired through good models of mental health in our parents, siblings, teachers, and associates. Positive mental health gives us the ability to assure that all these other areas are functioning well and to restore order in them if anything goes awry. Positive mental health, which includes a positive worldview, a can-do attitude, and care and concern for those around us, is thus the engine that makes life flow smoothly and without interruption. Positive mental health also includes a certain amount of good luck, or at least the expectation of good luck, and a belief that we can cope with whatever life has to offer.

If you arrive in old age blessed with positive mental health, great! If not, some of the things discussed in Chapters 3, 4, and 5, that is, finding your ideal place to live, staying socially connected, and doing and becoming exactly what you want to do and be, are building blocks to good mental health. So is your striving to maintain good physical health and to preserve or even increase your financial security. Other issues contributing to positive mental health are discussed throughout the book, especially in discussions on maintaining your brain, exercise, keeping your independence, inner and spiritual self, charitable giving, and how to say your final good-bye. The following story illustrates someone in my social circle who exemplifies positive mental health.

Nina just celebrated her 80th birthday. She is married to a man who is retired from being a minister. She has three children and five grandchildren. She was brought up in a somewhat privileged family as the daughter of a university professor, attended an Ivy League college and earned a master's degree in one of the social sciences. She spent most of her life as a minister's wife, herself ministering to many of her husband's parishioners who needed help. She experienced one tour in the Peace Corps in Africa and moved around several times as her husband served first one, then another congregation.

Nina now volunteers for her local elderly agency; participates in several university studies of brain function in old age; hosts innumerable social occasions for her children, grandchildren, their friends, and a large collection of other relatives. She belongs to a book club, attends exercise classes, lifts weights, walks regularly, and maintains a thin body. She frequently telephones her siblings, former classmates, and many friends, and she travels throughout the United States and to Europe, Mexico, and Canada several times a year.

She has had to cope with a son's multiple failed marriages, her husband's occasional depression, and the loss of both her parents and a brother, yet she remains positive and cheerful, although she can become quite exhausted from her many activities. She is "lightly spiritual," in that she generally supports the tenets of her husband's religion without being weighed down by any strict interpretation of that religious belief system. Her own health is good, although she takes medication for high blood pressure and low thyroid function under the supervision of a thoughtful primary care doctor. She enjoys a glass of wine with dinner nearly every night, but never drinks to excess. Watching her from a distance I have never known anyone to have been angry with her for any extended period of time. When asked for advice, she listens carefully and encourages people to deal with their problems head-on, never imposing her own views on the advice-seeker. Does Nina have good mental health? You be the judge.

The Relationship between Happiness and Mental Health

There is a close relationship between mental health and happiness, but the exact nature of this relationship is not entirely understood. Clearly, mentally ill persons are not happy—even the person in a manic phase of manic-depressive disease cannot be said to be happy, as consequences of his or her manic behavior will come to haunt the individual as soon as he/she leaves that phase. But are positive mental health and happiness one and the same? Probably not. Positive mental health is most likely the sturdier cousin in this relationship, as it requires many facets of behavior not required of someone who is "merely" happy. Happiness should be the prevailing mood, not the exception. Children generally appear to be happy, as are animals, unless they are deprived of their basic needs or if pain or threats are inflicted on them. So maintaining happiness throughout life probably requires relative freedom from deprivation, pain, and threats. On the positive side, maintaining a well-functioning social network (as discussed in Chapter 5), liking where you live (as discussed in Chapter 3), and a clear sense of self (as discussed in Chapter 4) are other factors contributing to happiness.

Mental Health Problems That Can Arise In Later Years

There are mental health problems which can arise in one's later years. This chapter will not cover mental health problems that began earlier in life and continue into old age but only those mental health problems that arise late in life. The most common of these are:

- Normal and abnormal grief reactions
- Clinically significant depression
- Anxiety disorders
- Alcohol abuse
- Addiction to pain medications

Normal and Abnormal Grief Reactions

Most people will probably experience one or more episodes of grief as they age. Grief is a normal, painful reaction to an important loss, especially the loss of a loved person. But grief can also be experienced over the loss of a job, of an ability, such as eyesight, or of a beloved pet. Grief is characterized by longing for a person or a thing that was lost and feelings of sadness, emptiness, and tearfulness. The resolution of grief requires time, usually weeks or months. It may include sharing one's feelings with relatives and trusted friends, and repeatedly recalling the virtues and values of the lost person, situation, thing, or pet. How much time it takes to resolve grief depends on a variety of factors: cultural patterns of grief resolution, the intensity of the lost relationship, the availability of social supports, and whether the loss can be replaced or restored.

Abnormal grief reactions are those that last longer than a few weeks or months. They may be caused by conflicted feelings about the lost relationship or by the absence of emotional support. Counseling by a professional grief counselor or a trained therapist may be needed. Medication, such as an antidepressant, is generally not needed, however, unless a full-blown depression develops, which is discussed below.

Sometimes grieving can precede the actual death of the individual, such as with the occurrence of Alzheimer's disease in a loved one, where the loss of companionship and support precedes actual death by months or years. When death eventually comes, the finality of the loss may lead to a new episode of grief. Because the eventual death is often accompanied by a sense of relief when the suffering is finally over, this may lead to a new problem: the bereaved individual feels guilty over the sense of relief. Again, individual or group counseling can help to clarify that a sense of relief is normal and understandable and not a cause for self-flagellation.

Clinically Significant Depression

Depression is by far the most common emotional problem to occur in older people. Most of us know what depression looks and feels like: it's a persistent state of deep sadness, not merely the occasional episode of the blues, which is normal for any of us to experience.

Clinically significant depression is characterized by persistent sadness, tearfulness, pervasive pessimism and negativism, low energy, and a loss of interest in one's usual activities, including decreased appetite and resulting weight loss. The depressed individual usually speaks with a low, monotonous voice, shows a slumped posture, has difficulty falling asleep and staying asleep, and often loses interest in sexual activity. Moreover, the depressed person is usually unable to carry on their regular occupational and social activities. Feelings of hopelessness may be expressed, and suicidal ideas or even suicide attempts may occur. For all these reasons, it is clear that *clinically significant depression requires treatment.* What causes or triggers depression? Most commonly, depression sets in after a person sustains one or more significant losses that dim the individual's view of the future. Sometimes depression occurs after lengthy periods of extreme stress, such as that experienced by a person in a demanding caregiver role. Sometimes it is a response to disappointment over one's children's prospects, or any other situation for which the person feels there is no possible solution. In addition to life events, depression may also occur for biologic or genetic reasons, without an external precipitating event.

Treatment of depression optimally consists of both psychological and medical intervention. A depressed person needs counseling with a trained therapist who can discuss alternative solutions and antidepressant medication. Those who are actively suicidal may need to be hospitalized, or at a minimum be under the constant supervision of a responsible family member or friend. The prognosis for treatment of depression is often good. Most people can either fully recover or at least improve markedly in their functioning. Persons who have experienced one episode of clinical depression are at greater risk for a recurrence of depression. For this reason they may need to continue on antidepressant medication, as well as continue with counseling or psychotherapy.

Anxiety Disorders

Here I am talking about a state of continued anxiety, not the occasional bit of anxiety that vexes everyone from time to time when things threaten to go wrong. Fearfulness, excessive worrying, and social timidity may be accompanied by physical symptoms such as heart palpitations or excessive sweating of the hands. Sometimes persons with anxiety reactions can experience frank panic attacks, which can be very upsetting and paralyzing. Psychotherapy and counseling, aimed at finding alternative reactions to the feared situation, are indicated. This approach can then also be combined with the judicious use of anti-anxiety medications, which are effective in alleviating both the psychological as well as the physical manifestations of anxiety.

Alcohol Abuse

For a variety of reasons, the abuse of alcohol has become a significant problem to a sizeable number of persons in their later years. One cause for this is the relatively frequent occurrence of losses, disappointments, medical problems, social isolation, boredom, and other adverse events in this age group. Another cause is inherent in the nature of alcohol itself. Used in moderation, it is relaxing, serves as a social lubricant, and is readily available. But regular use of more than a few drinks a day, more than a few times a week, can become a problem in itself. It can lead to further social isolation, to accidents, to poorer management of medical conditions, to decreased productivity, disturbed sleep, and even to malnutrition. Importantly, as one ages, the impact of a single drink is almost double that of such a drink in younger years, due to changed metabolism in the aging individual. Accordingly, for anyone who has come to abuse alcohol in one's later years, total abstinence is probably the only solution. This can be accomplished by an individual's personal decision, a firm medical recommendation, or though group support like that provided by Alcoholics Anonymous. The contributing mental, social, and medical problems need to be addressed through means other than the use of alcohol.

Addiction to Pain Medications

Aging individuals may also be at increased risk for addiction to pain medications. Because pain syndromes, such as arthritis, diabetic neuropathy, or post-shingles pain, are relatively common in the later years, pain medication is often prescribed for older individuals. Given that they alleviate physical pain, they may also be used to alleviate mental pain and discomfort to the person's detriment. With the exception of aspirin, acetaminophen, and non-steroidal anti-inflammatory agents, most of the other frequently prescribed pain medications are both habit-forming and prone to drug tolerance. Drug tolerance means that, over time, increasing dosages are required to give the same amount of pain relief. An additional risk factor leading to addiction to pain medication is when a person is receiving pain medications from more than one physician or specialist, such as a surgeon, a rheumatologist, and a pain specialist, each being unaware of another physician prescribing similar pain medication.

Accordingly, the primary care physician should strictly supervise all of the person's pain medications to avoid potential abuse and addiction. Once addiction to pain medication has been developed and recognized, a systematic withdrawal program under an experienced addiction specialist needs to be carried out. An exception to the concern about addiction to pain medication is the individual receiving pain medications for cancer pain under a hospice care physician.

Some Unique Features of Treating Mental Health Problems

There are several unique features related to the treatment of mental health problems that need to be discussed:

- Health insurance coverage for mental health problems differs from insurance coverage for physical health problems.

- Participation in mental health treatment is never just a passive process.
- There is a need to distinguish between the various health professionals offering mental health treatments: psychiatrists, psychologists, social workers, and mental health counselors.

Health Insurance Coverage for Mental Health Problems Differs from Coverage for Physical Health Problems

Until recently, treatment for emotional disorders was not always covered by medical insurance. Some policies provided no such coverage, while others severely limited the amount of care paid for by insurance, or required high co-payments for such care. Even Medicare has shown this same prejudice against mental health care: Medicare generally pays 80 percent of the cost of medical procedures, but pays only 50 percent for mental health treatments. Increasingly, new legislation is mandating equal coverage of emotional or psychological problems on par with that for physical problems. But this is not yet uniformly so. You, as a consumer, need to know exactly what kind of mental health care coverage your policy provides. Recent efforts at health care reform have sought to require parity for mental health services on a national level. At the time of this writing, the outcome of these efforts is not yet certain.

Mental Health Treatment Is Never Just a Passive Process

Sometimes humor can illuminate an issue: "How many psychiatrists does it take to change a light bulb?" The answer is: "Only one, but the light bulb must really want to change."

The point made is that psychological or mental health treatment always requires the active involvement of the affected individual. Real improvement cannot be simply administered by someone, as it might in the treatment of some physical disorders. But even in regard to physical health care, I have already advised that you need to be actively involved in your own care, that is, you need to be your own health care manager. This is all the more true in bringing about psychological change. You must take responsibility for maintaining and restoring your own mental health, with the assistance of professional mental health care providers.

Distinguishing between Various Mental Health Care Providers

A few words about the players involved in providing mental health services:

PSYCHIATRISTS

Psychiatrists are physicians who have been especially trained to recognize and treat emotional as well as physical disorders. Because older patients often have both physical as well as emotional disorders, there is some advantage to being under the care of someone who understands and can treat physical problems as well. Also, psychiatrists can prescribe medications, such as antidepressant or anti-anxiety medications.

PSYCHOLOGISTS

Psychologists are mental health professionals trained in recognizing and treating mental but not physical disorders. They may provide counseling and psychotherapy, but they are not authorized to prescribe medications. They are not necessarily more or less competent than psychiatrists in providing such counseling.

SOCIAL WORKERS

Social workers most commonly hold a master's degree and are trained in knowing community resources and family structure, understanding emotional disorders, and providing counseling or psychotherapy. They may be particularly valuable when family or community issues are involved.

MENTAL HEALTH COUNSELORS

Mental health counselors are yet another group of professionals sometimes involved in providing mental health care, but their training and licensing varies greatly from state to state.

Each of these types of mental health professionals can play a significant role in providing mental services, depending on the specific aspects of any given mental health problem.

CHAPTER SUMMARY

- There is no health without mental health.
- Understand and achieve optimal mental health.
- Understand and receive treatment for any mental or emotional problems that may occur.
- Understand that health insurance coverage for mental health problems may differ from coverage provided for physical health problems.
- Your participation in any mental health treatment needs to be an active, not a passive, affair.
- Understand the differing characteristics and qualifications of various mental health care providers.

Chapter 8

Care for Your Brain to Keep Your Memory Sharp

WHEN I FIRST came to the University of South Florida to start a program on aging, I asked hundreds of people what they feared most about growing old. Most often they replied that they feared losing their memory, their mental capacity, and their ability to make decisions. It wasn't heart disease or stroke or cancer that most scared them: it was fear of losing their mind, their brain power. One woman of my acquaintance expressed this sentiment particularly powerfully:

> Laura, age 67, developed an illness that her local doctors could not easily diagnose. She had abdominal pain and weight loss, and felt fatigued all the time. They referred her to the Mayo

Clinic in Rochester, Minnesota, for a complete workup. After several days of extensive testing, the doctors at Mayo were able to make a definitive diagnosis: they told her that she had cancer of the pancreas, that surgery for the condition was virtually impossible, and that in all likelihood she would not recover. She returned home and confided to her best friend, "At least now I know what it is. Thank God, it's not Alzheimer's."

Hearing sentiments like this contributed greatly to our choosing Alzheimer's disease and related memory disorders as our number one priority at the Suncoast Gerontology Center, and it's also why this book devotes considerable attention to issues related to memory. The first part of this chapter covers how memory problems can be recognized, how they can be prevented, and what treatment options are available. In the second part, I share my best tips, secrets, and exercises for how to maintain your brain at its highest level of functioning.

Types of Memory Loss

Four types of memory problems exist in old age: benign forgetfulness, minor cognitive impairment, Alzheimer's disease, and other forms of dementia.

Benign Forgetfulness

Benign forgetfulness happens to the *majority* of people over age 65. It is annoying but not serious. Benign forgetfulness is characterized by relatively minor slowing of your memory capacity and manifests itself in a number of little ways, such as forgetting where you parked your car, or recognizing someone at a social gathering but being unable to recall their name right then and there. (A little while later the name comes back to you, and you feel somewhat foolish.) Or, it may be a matter of having more difficulty in learning new information: learning how to operate new gadgets or remembering new phone numbers may not be as easy as it was years ago.

With a little extra concentration, you can usually overcome these problems. You may need to write down new information; you may need to make associations between familiar names or words with an unfamiliar word or name you are trying to learn in order to better remember it. You may need to have someone show you more than once how your new smartphone or DVD player works. But you can still learn. You can still remember. You may just have to work a little harder. You may need to write yourself more notes: jot down the aisle number where you parked your car, or *always* place your house keys, your purse, or your wallet in exactly the same spot every time you come into the house. The good news about benign forgetfulness is that it doesn't get any worse, and it does not lead to Alzheimer's disease. The bad news is that it doesn't get any better either. You need to understand it, accept it, and deal with it in ways like those mentioned above.

Minor Cognitive Impairment

Minor memory impairment, or more formally *minor cognitive impairment,* is serious, but not fatal. Minor cognitive impairment is characterized by completely forgetting whole sequences of events in which you have actively participated. This can be embarrassing, or worse. For instance:

John, age 70, lives in Florida and regularly attends an annual family reunion in Tennessee. Last year, when he came back, his son-in-law asked him about the reunion. John said he had not attended at all. But his daughter, who also attended, had recorded a videotape of the reunion. When John saw the video, showing him clearly participating and interacting at the event, he broke into tears. He realized fully for the first time that he had completely forgotten about the event. He also realized the implications of the occurrence: his memory problems were greater than mere absentmindedness.

What happens in minor cognitive impairment is that the brain participates in the actual experience, but no memory trace is laid down. It is somewhat like not pressing the "enter" or the "save" button on your computer. If such a situation occurs more than once or twice, you should undergo a thorough memory evaluation by a specialist in memory disorders, someone beyond your primary care doctor. This could be a psychiatrist, a neurologist, or an internist, but, in any case, it should be a doctor who has a strong interest and extensive experience in memory evaluations. Standard memory tests may need to be performed. In addition, your ability for *delayed recall* of information may need to be tested. Delayed recall of new information is one of the earliest signs of minor cognitive impairment. Further evaluation may require a session with a trained neuropsychologist, an MRI (magnetic resonance imaging), or a PET (positron emission tomography) scan. An MRI is a test that produces an actual image of the brain, and it can pick up early indications of brain cell loss. A PET scan is similar but even more specialized and expensive, and it can pick up changes in brain cell activity or metabolism before there is any loss of brain tissue.

If you or someone close to you is diagnosed with minor cognitive impairment, it can and should be treated by a memory specialist. Medications that have been approved for the treatment of Alzheimer's disease, such as Aricept, Exelon, or Razadyne, have been shown to also be of benefit to persons with minor cognitive impairment. While minor cognitive impairment isn't yet Alzheimer's dementia, it may well be the earliest stage of Alzheimer's disease.

Alzheimer's Disease

Alzheimer's disease, on the other hand, is a problem of an entirely different magnitude. First of all, it is a disease of the brain, not merely a manifestation of aging. It is a disease in which brain cells die prematurely and progressively. This leaves an individual with impaired memory function, impaired decision-making ability, and reduced reasoning and learning capacity.

The symptoms vary wildly, and the disease can last anywhere from 2 to more than 20 years, eventually resulting in death, unless the person dies from another illness before then. President Ronald Reagan, for instance, lived with Alzheimer's disease for 17 years.

In some individuals, Alzheimer's is primarily characterized by increasing degrees of memory and intellectual decline. Others with Alzheimer's may also exhibit behavioral problems, which can often be more vexing to the caregiver than memory problems. Behavioral problems can include depression, agitation, irritability, hostility, and even hallucinations and delusions. It is one thing to care for a nice little old lady who is a bit forgetful but otherwise pleasant, and quite another to deal with someone who is hostile, suspicious, aggressive, or fears that the caregiver is trying to poison him or her.

Thus it is not surprising that Alzheimer's disease is sometimes referred to as "the big A" by patients and family members. It can indeed be a devastating disorder. When it is suspected, it urgently requires prompt diagnosis, followed immediately by treatment in order to preserve memory and intellectual capacity at the highest level for as long as possible. When Alzheimer's disease strikes, it has at least two victims: the person with the disease and the people who become caregivers of the person with the disease. Caregivers might be a spouse, an adult child, a son-or daughter-in-law, a close friend, or several of these. A person without a family caregiver may need to have paid caregivers and/or a professional care manager. Later in this chapter there are some practical tips and advice for caregivers.

Here are the seven warnings signs of Alzheimer's disease. I developed this list at the Suncoast Alzheimer's and Gerontology Center at the University of South Florida. The purpose of this list is to alert laypersons and professionals to the early warning signs of one of the most devastating disorders affecting older people—Alzheimer's disease. If someone has several of these symptoms, it does not mean that they definitely have the disease. It does mean that they should be thoroughly examined by a medical specialist trained in evaluating memory disorders, such as a neurologist or a psychiatrist, or by a comprehensive memory disorder clinic, with an entire team of experts knowledgeable about memory problems. A person who has four or more of these signs is very likely to suffer from either Alzheimer's disease or from a dementia due to other causes.

THE SEVEN WARNING SIGNS OF ALZHEIMER'S DISEASE

1. Asking the same question over and over again.
2. Repeating the same story, word for word, again and again.
3. Forgetting how to do activities that were previously done with ease and regularity, such as cooking or playing cards.
4. Losing one's ability to pay bills or balance one's checkbook.
5. Getting lost in familiar surroundings, or misplacing household objects.
6. Neglecting to bathe or wearing the same clothes over and over again, while insisting that they have taken a bath or that their clothes are still clean.
7. Relying on someone else, such as a spouse, to make decisions or answer questions they previously would have handled themselves.

Dementia is defined as a memory disorder due to the loss of brain cells. Causes of dementia other than Alzheimer's disease may include a major stroke or multiple smaller strokes, multiple brain traumas, chronic alcoholism, or a history of encephalitis. Dementia can also occur in the late stages of Parkinson's disease or as the result of Lewy Body disease, a variant of Alzheimer's disease.

If your attempts to identify these seven signs of Alzheimer's do not sufficiently indicate whether a problem exists, and you are still concerned about a family member or friend, there is another test available. I developed the Short Portable Mental Status Questionnaire (see figure on facing page) to measure the presence and the degree of memory loss. The questionnaire is usually administered by a doctor, nurse, or social worker, but a layperson can do it as well.

Accordingly, *you* could ask someone about whose memory you are concerned these questions to determine if they are experiencing significant memory loss. Please note that this is not a self-administered test. It allows the examiner to determine if the person's memory is normal, or whether he or she has mild, moderate, or severe memory loss, according to the scale shown on the next page. However, it will not allow you to make a definite diagnosis of Alzheimer's disease or other memory disorder. If there is evidence of significant memory loss, a full medical evaluation should be arranged as soon as possible.

Until the early 1990s, doctors said that you couldn't definitively diagnose Alzheimer's disease until a brain autopsy had been performed. Sure, this made for an ac-

	PFEIFFER
SPMSQ	**SHORT PORTABLE MENTAL STATUS QUESTIONNAIRE**

INSTRUCTIONS: Ask the subject questions 1-10, record answer, and enter as "1" under appropriate column (correct/error). All responses, to be scored correct, must be given by subject without reference to calendar, newspaper, birth certificate or other memory aid.	Patient Name: _____ Date: _____

		CORRECT	ERROR
1.	WHAT IS THE DATE TODAY? Month_____ Day_____ Year_____ (Score correct only when the exact month, day and year are given correctly.)		
2.	WHAT DAY OF THE WEEK IS IT? Day_____		
3.	WHAT IS THE NAME OF THIS PLACE? _____ (Score correct if any correct description of the location is given: "My home," accurate name of town, city or name of residence, hospital, or institution (if subject is institutionalized) are all acceptable.)		
4.	WHAT IS YOUR TELEPHONE NUMBER? (If none see 4A below) (Score correct when the correct number can be verified or when subject can repeat the same number at another point in question.) #_____ 4A. WHAT IS YOUR STREET ADDRESS? (Ask only if subject does not have a telephone.) _____		
5.	HOW OLD ARE YOU? AGE:_____ (Score correct when stated age corresponds to date of birth.)		
6.	WHEN WERE YOU BORN? Month_____ Day_____ Year_____ (Score correct only when exact month, date, and year are all given.)		
7.	WHO IS PRESIDENT OF THE UNITED STATES NOW?_____ (Only the last name of the President is required.)		
8.	WHO WAS THE PRESIDENT BEFORE HIM?_____ (Only the last name of the previous President is required.)		
9.	WHAT WAS YOUR MOTHER'S MAIDEN NAME?_____ (Does not need to be verified. Score correct if a female name plus last name other than subject's is given.)		
10.	SUBRACT 3 FROM 20 AND KEEP SUBTRACTING 3 FROM EACH NEW NUMBER ALL THE WAY DOWN. ___ ___ ___ ___ ___ ___ (The entire series must be performed correctly in order to be scored correct. Any error in series or unwillingness to attempt series is scored as incorrect.)		

TOTAL NUMBER OF ERRORS

*ADJUSTMENT FACTOR

A)   SUBTRACT 1 FROM ERROR SCORE IF SUBJECT HAS HAD ONLY A GRADE SCHOOL EDUCATION   -

B)   ADD 1 TO ERROR SCORE IF SUBJECT HAS HAD EDUCATION BEYOND HIGH SCHOOL   +

TOTAL ADJUSTED ERRORS

SCORING KEY: 0-2 errors = intellectually intact; 3-4 errors = mildly impaired; 5-7 errors = moderately impaired; 8-10 errors = severely impaired.

INFORMATION OBTAINED BY:	DATE:

curate diagnosis, but, unfortunately, it was too late to do the patient or the caregiver any good. Today, we are able to diagnose Alzheimer's disease at every stage of the disease—mild, moderate, or severe—with 90 to 95 percent certainty.

Also, until the early 1990s, there was *no treatment* for Alzheimer's disease. Again, real progress has been made in this area as well, and Alzheimer's disease is now a treatable disorder. The currently available treatments do not cure the disease, but they can slow its progression. Therefore, it is extremely important that the diagnosis be made as early as possible, and that treatment be started immediately after the diagnosis. Early treatment brings the best chance of retaining maximum functioning capacity in the affected individual and eases the burden of care on the family caregiver.

Treating Alzheimer's Disease

There are now several medications available for the treatment of Alzheimer's disease. The current standard of treatment involves the use of Namenda *in combination* with one of the three other drugs: Aricept, Exelon, or Razadyne. The *combination* of Namenda with one of these drugs has an *additive,* or greater, benefit than if any one these drugs is used alone. Treatment with these drugs should be started as soon as the diagnosis is made, and should be continued until late into the disease, as these drugs continue to slow the rate of progression of both memory and behavioral problems. Additional medications are being tested that may bring about even greater benefits than the current medications, so it is important to pay attention when additional medications for the treatment of Alzheimer's disease become available.

Manuel was a successful businessman, community leader, and philanthropist. He and his wife, Cathy, were very close. They went everywhere together. At age 70, Cathy began to repeat herself incessantly; she often misplaced her keys, lost her checkbook, and needed to be reminded about her appointments. At first, Manuel tried to rationalize Cathy's forgetfulness and hide his concern about her from friends and family members. He didn't want to believe that she could possibly be developing Alzheimer's disease. However, as her symptoms continued to worsen, he became sufficiently concerned that he sought professional help. Cathy was evaluated, and doctors told Manuel that she did indeed have Alzheimer's disease. Cathy was quickly started on treatment. Early on, her doctor advised Manuel that he should consider seeking help with caring for his wife, but he insisted that he would be the only one to look after her. Both he and Cathy were very private people, and neither one wanted to accept the idea of a stranger coming into their home.

As Cathy became more and more impaired, and Manuel had to do more and more for her, he became increasingly depressed, but he still refused to get any help with his caregiving duties. Cathy got up several times during the night, was agitated, and Manuel got very little sleep. Still, he insisted that he do everything for her, and that no one else could care for Cathy as well as he could. Then, within 24 hours, two things happened: Cathy got up in the middle of the night and fell in the bathroom, injuring her chest and head. Manuel himself injured his back trying to lift her from the bathroom floor. He finally called his daughter and allowed her to bring in live-in help for both of them. A few weeks later he confessed to Cathy's doctor, "I'm so relieved we have help now. I should have listened to your advice a lot sooner."

As mentioned earlier, Alzheimer's disease has two victims: the patient and the family caregiver. At times it is difficult to say which of the two suffers more or has the harder job. If you are thrust into the role of a care-giver, you have two main responsibilities—one toward the patient and one toward yourself. Caregivers must take on an ever-increasing series of tasks for their loved one, while what they need to do for themselves is similarly demanding and important.

The caregiver essentially becomes the patient's guardian angel, using a caring, alert, and supervisory approach. This means letting the patient do everything he or she can do, while being ready to assist with anything that person can no longer do. Caregivers take patients to the doctor, handle their legal and financial affairs, and take them shopping or on an outing. Yes, they become their loved one's chauffeur, since patients with all but mild Alzheimer's should not drive any more.

Other Forms of Dementia

A number of other dementias also exist. These include vascular, Lewy Body, post-traumatic, and post-encephalitic dementias. Differentiating between the various types of dementia should be left to your memory doctor. Treatments may differ for some of these other dementias, but they can include similar elements, such as the use of one or more of the anti-Alzheimer's drugs. Many of the aspects of caring for someone with another form of dementia are similar to those found in caring for an Alzheimer's patient. If you or your loved one is dealing with one or another of these dementias, look for a book written for people dealing with that specific form of dementia.

Take Care of Yourself

As a caregiver, you must also take care of yourself. You need to preserve and protect yourself, so that you do not wear out, burn out, or otherwise become disabled. You need to have your own needs met, to attend to your personal care, your medical care, your financial dealings, and so on. You will need to take some time for yourself, away from the patient. It is important to find someone who can assist you in the care of the patient for a few hours, a few days a week, or whatever length of time you need to get your own mental and physical health needs met. You cannot afford to be consumed by the caregiving experience. You will need to share the burden of care with someone else, especially in the later stages of the patient's disease. People are often hesitant to ask for help but be assured that such help is absolutely necessary, for your own good and for that of your loved one. One of the most powerful phrases in the human language is, "I need your help." Use that phrase. You will seldom be turned down. And, as is illustrated in the story about Manuel and Cathy, it's important to do so earlier rather than later.

The Art of Caregiving

Here are a few other things you should do if you become the caregiver of an Alzheimer's patient. Read *The Thirty-Six Hour Day* by Nancy Mace and Peter Rabins. It is readily available at your local library or bookstore. Join a support group to learn how other caregivers cope with caregiving tasks. You may also be able to help other caregivers by sharing what you have learned about caregiving and that could be a source of added self-esteem. And get help with your caregiving duties from family members and friends, or employ someone who has been trained to assist in the care of the memory-impaired. Your local area Agency on Aging, which exists in every sizeable community, or your Visiting Nurse Associations can help you find someone qualified. However, your primary care doctor may need to write you a prescription for you to receive VNA services.

Maintain Your Brain

Having covered the various memory problems—serious ones and not so serious ones—let's now discuss how to *maintain your brain* in its optimal, healthiest state. I am going to address three specific topics:

- How to exercise your brain
- How to feed your brain
- How to protect your brain

First, here's a story that illustrates some of the points made in this section:

Andrea's mother had died of Alzheimer's disease. Andrea had cared for her, initially by long distance. Eventually, when her mother needed nursing home care, Andrea moved her to a nursing home near her so that she could keep an eye on her mother and on her mother's care. After her mother's death, Andrea decided to do everything she could to avoid falling victim to her mother's disease. She read voraciously, consulted with experts, scoured the Internet for information, and tried to do everything she could to maintain her brain. Andrea took a dance class to learn basic ballet steps and regularly participated with friends in line dancing, which provided vigorous exercise. She ate sparingly, emphasizing fruits and vegetables, tried to approximate a Mediterranean diet, and drank one glass of red wine every day. As a widow, she felt liberated to do many things in the community. She started a play-reading group at her home and contributed to many charitable organizations. At age 75, her community honored her as "Woman of the Year." She took a number of vitamins and supplements as well as fish-oil capsules on a regular basis. She had read that falls were a particular danger to older people, and she purchased and read *How to Prevent Falls* by Betty Perkins Carpenter and gave copies of the book to a few of her older friends. She is enjoying life and so far has escaped any signs of Alzheimer's disease.

Your brain is the most important—and the most precious—organ in your body. It doesn't just control your memory and your thoughts; it also controls your emotions, your movements, and your "inner milieu," that is, your hormonal balance. It is the seat of your sense of self and your self-esteem. It is your interface with the world.

In order to maintain your brain, you need to exercise it, you need to feed it, and you need to protect it from harm, as Andrea did. Let us consider these strategies one at a time.

Exercise Your Brain

Your brain is not a muscle, but in many ways it acts like a muscle, yet is infinitely more complex. Like a muscle, you must use it regularly in order to maintain its "strength"; it is a "use-it-or-lose-it" proposition. Contrary to the old saying, "You can't teach an old dog new tricks," the aging brain actually *thrives* on new information, new skills, and new challenges. It is also important to refresh old skills and information, but that is less important than acquiring new ones.

There are many ways to "exercise" your brain. Accordingly, you have many types of activities to choose from. Here are some possibilities, although the list is endless: learn a new language, learn new dance steps, learn the art of tai chi, become familiar with surfing the Internet, and read books, both fiction and non-fiction, on subjects that interest you. Also, read newspapers and magazines (although I would avoid spending too much time on all the trouble spots in the world—that can be just too depressing). Engage in conversations with others on a regular basis, start a new hobby, such as photography, or start a new business. Any of these "exercises" can be very challenging to your brain.

And now a word about doing puzzles. The kind of puzzles that require new skills and new information benefit your brain greatly. Puzzles that rely primarily on information you already have, such as crossword puzzles, which rely primarily on the vocabulary you already possess, are less helpful, unless you make solving crossword puzzles a social, competitive occasion. Doing crossword puzzles by yourself may lead to social isolation. (Sorry to throw cold water on what may be one of your favorite activities.) It doesn't hurt, but, by itself, it doesn't help much. People with quite advanced Alzheimer's disease often amaze their relatives by doing crossword puzzles, because they rely on long-ago established skills, not on new intellectual or current challenges.

Feed Your Brain

What do I mean by "feed your brain"? Your brain needs glucose and oxygen. These are provided by the blood that flows through your brain. You need to work with your doctor to assure that blood flow is ample, steady, and uninterrupted. This means that you must do everything you can to avoid clogged arteries, high blood pressure, or low blood pressure. Specifically, know your cholesterol numbers: keep total cholesterol below 200 (or whatever number your doctor recommends), and keep your high-density cholesterol (HDL), the so-called "good cholesterol," above 50. Treat high blood pressure to reduce the risk of stroke. Monitor for low blood pressure, as treatment for high blood pressure can sometimes overshoot the goal. Low blood pressure reduces blood flow to the brain. If you have diabetes, a common disease in the elderly, treat it so that your blood sugar levels remain normal or near normal. Treat chronic pulmonary disease so that blood oxygen levels are not lowered. Treat any heartbeat irregularities, since these can interrupt blood supply to the brain.

Most importantly, get regular exercise, which is explored in detail in Chapter 10. Also, you need to get an adequate supply of vitamins and minerals. At a minimum, take a "senior" multi-vitamin capsule every day, and also take one or two 1,000-mg capsules of fish oil, containing both EPA (eicosapentaenoic) and DHA (docosahexaenoic acid) omega-3 fatty acids each day. Some older individuals can tolerate only one capsule of fish oil per day, as a higher dose may cause easy bruising of the skin. Read the discussion on vitamins, minerals, hormones, and supplements in the Appendix for further details.

Finally, get enough rest. Sleep is the great restorer. Make every effort to get seven to eight hours of sleep each night. It will help your brain recover from all the activities of your day. In order to be able to sleep seven to eight hours a night, go to sleep at the same time each night. Get plenty of exercise during the day so that you will feel tired at night. Avoid coffee or caffeine-containing soft drinks after midday and develop some type of relaxation technique for just before bedtime.

Protect Your Brain

What do I mean by "protect your brain"? For one thing, do not expose your brain to any head trauma. This means taking care to avoid falls: remove slippery rugs in your home, install handrails in the bathroom, and, for those of you living up north, avoid going out on icy sidewalks. Falls are extremely dangerous to the elderly. In addition to concussions or even brain hemorrhages, they can lead to hip fractures requiring bed rest and extensive rehabilitation. In case you should fall, have yourself evaluated in an emergency room.

Protect your brain from excessive use of alcohol; avoid more than one alcoholic drink per day as your brain is now much more sensitive to the effect of alcohol. You will also want to avoid excessive medications, particularly any that induce drowsiness. But first check with your doctor who could provide a non-drowsiness producing alternative.

Also, make sure your doctor is aware of all over-the-counter medications and supplements you take. In addition, get into the habit of reading about potential side effects of medications or supplements you take and report to your doctor any such side effect that you experience. Your doctor may be able to take you off of the offending medication altogether, or switch to one that does not produce drowsiness. Make sure you actively treat, or get treatment for, any acute illnesses. Illnesses that cause fever can cloud mental and memory functions significantly.

So there you are. Treat your brain like it was your most precious and fragile possession. It is, and you need to rely on it for everything else you want to do in all the years to come. Taking care of your brain can be fun, from tango lessons to trigonometry to travels to Timbuktu.

Chapter Summary

- Memory really matters.
- Understand benign forgetfulness.
- Understand minor cognitive impairment.
- Understand Alzheimer's disease.
- Understand other dementias.
- Maintain your brain.
- Feed your brain.
- Exercise your brain.
- Protect your brain.
- Review *The Seven Warning Signs of Alzheimer's Disease and the Short Portable Mental Status Questionnaire* included in this chapter. These are of particular value in understanding memory problems.

Chapter 9

Hold On to Your Money
So You Don't Outlive It

This chapter was co-authored by Terri Gaffney, JD, LLM in taxation (General Counsel, Overstreet Wealth Management, Inc., Tampa, Florida).

THIS CHAPTER deals with retirement income: how to determine if you have enough; how to preserve it; how to increase it, if necessary; and how to guard against any losses through scams or other deceptive practices. A stable stream of income is an essential element of successful aging. It makes possible everything that is needed in retirement: suitable housing, adequate medical care, entertainment, and gift-giving to family members and to charity. The topic of money is not only important, it is also very intriguing and stimulating.

For starters, you might as well accept the fact that you are not suddenly going to get rich in your later years: those from whom you might have inherited money or property have probably already passed away, and the likelihood that you will win the lottery is remote. Accordingly, the level of your income during your working years will almost certainly define your income level in retirement. For the majority of us, that will be slightly less than your earnings during your working years, somewhere between one-half and two-thirds of your previous earnings. For most people that will be adequate, barring unforeseen or catastrophic circumstances. But catastrophic circumstances can occur, as we saw in 2008, when the United States and the world economy imploded.

Three Kinds of Money

For our purposes here, it may be useful to think of your money in three categories. The first category is money that you, or you and your partner, cannot outlive, and which is guaranteed. It may be guaranteed by the integrity and/or rating of an insurance company, by your former employer, such as a state or a corporation, or by the full faith and credit of the government of the United States. This kind of money can also be expected to be paid to you on a regular basis, either monthly, quarterly, semi-annually, or annually. The second category is money that is not guaranteed, that you can outlive, but which you can also pass on to your heirs if you do not consume it all during your lifetime. The third category is new money, or income that you earn during your retirement.

Money That You Cannot Outlive

The advantage of this kind of money is that *you* can determine how it will be distributed: over your lifetime, or over the lifetime of you and your partner. The downside of this kind of money is that in the normal course there will not be any remainder of that money to pass on to your children, to your estate, or to charity. It is very important that you have enough money in this first category to carry you and your partner comfortably through all of your later years.

Money that is guaranteed and that you cannot outlive includes:

- Your Social Security income
- Your pension income, if any
- Some types of annuity income

SOCIAL SECURITY

For the vast majority of older Americans, Social Security will be the most basic source of income though not necessarily the largest one. The best part of Social Security income is that *it will last as long as you do.* For a married couple, when one of you dies, the survivor will continue to receive the majority of his or her previous benefits. Social Security even has a significant cost-of-living increase built into it, which may at least partially offset increasing costs and inflation.

Social Security also makes you eligible for Medicare coverage, which is your basic health care coverage in retirement.

However, for most people, Social Security income alone and Medicare health insurance alone is not enough, and you will need other sources of income as well as additional health care coverage.

PENSIONS

Significant numbers of elderly individuals are also going to be covered by a pension plan through their employer. Pension plans vary enormously, from minimal to very generous. They are provided by an employer to employees, as a contractual obligation of their employment and are proportional to the length of employment. If you are eligible for a pension, you typically know ahead of time what you will receive in the way of a pension. Most pensions have a variety of options available to the recipient. The highest level of payout generally applies if it continues only for the life of the one person covered by the pension. Somewhat reduced levels of payout are available if you want the pension to last not only for your own life but also for that of your beneficiary, such as your spouse or partner. If you wish to have your pension paid over the life of two people, you can make an additional choice: You can be paid a larger amount if you are willing to have the payment reduced to two-thirds for the survivor when one of you dies; a smaller amount will be paid out if you want the survivor to receive the same amount as when both of you were living. I strongly recommend that you choose an option that continues the payment of the pension to both you and your survivor.

ANNUITIES

An annuity is a contract sold by an insurance company designed to provide payment to the holder, usually on a monthly basis, from the designated start date to the end of the annuitant's and/or the co-annuitant's (usually spouse's) life. Broadly speaking, there are two types of annuity products: fixed annuities and variable annuities. Fixed annuities are not investment products (that is, there is no risk of losing the original principal sum), while variable annuities are investment products and could potentially result in losing your investment. With respect to fixed-annuity products, there are a number of variations referred to: Single Premium Immediate Annuities, Equity Indexed Deferred Annuities, and Straight Deferred Annuities. All of the above-mentioned fixed annuities require the deposit of a certain sum of money with an insurance company for the purchase of a specific annuity product. Depending on the specific product you purchase, you will receive options and/or guarantees that may include periodic payments for a specific amount of time, periodic payments for the life of the annuitant, or periodic payments for the life of the annuitant and the spouse or partner of the annuitant. Annuities are sold by insurance companies, and, as noted above, there are many variations to consider when purchasing an annuity. (Sometimes, life insurance products can also be used for retirement planning, but the intricacies of using them as a source of retirement income is beyond the scope of this discussion.)

With respect to variable annuities, it is best to remember that, unlike fixed annuities, there is a possibility of loss associated with this kind of annuity. There are variable annuity products available on the markets that claim to dampen the risk of loss, if purchased carefully with the assistance of a knowledgeable professional. For the purpose of the discussion at hand, it is probably best to eliminate variable annuities from the list of options that meet the safety requirements set out earlier. In short, *variable annuities are generally to be avoided in retirement.*

A fixed annuity can be based on an equity index which allows for some possible growth, or it can be a straight annuity in which the amounts paid out are fixed at the beginning of the contract. A fixed annuity can also begin immediately, based on a single premium purchase, or it can be paid out on a deferred basis, starting at an age specified by the purchaser of the annuity. You can determine whether the payout will cover only you for your lifetime or cover both you and your partner for both of your lifetimes. You should review the suitability of an annuity by reviewing sample annuities presented to you by an insurance company. It might also be a good idea to have any annuity you are considering for purchase reviewed by your financial advisor. The terms, methods of payout, and duration of payment should be accorded the greatest scrutiny prior to the purchase of the annuity.

CHARITABLE REMAINDER TRUST

Another vehicle for assuring income during retirement is a charitable remainder trust. This is an arrangement whereby assets, either real property, cash, or cash equivalents, are donated to a charity. The donor, who is also the grantor of the charitable remainder trust, receives income for a period of time or for his or her life, depending on how the charitable remainder trust is structured. At the death of the donor, the charity receives the residual trust assets. The donor avoids capital gains tax on the assets under current IRS regulations. Further, the donor may receive a charitable income tax deduction. The charitable remainder trust, which is irrevocable, is a highly complex trust that one should create only with the assistance of an attorney with significant experience in the areas of trust creation, charitable remainder trusts, and taxation.

Another fascinating aspect of your guaranteed money is that the longer you (and your co-annuitant) manage to live, the greater the total amount of money you will be able to receive over your lifetime(s). So from that point of view, you want to remain as healthy as possible for as long as possible so that you can be a winner in this regard as well. You've already paid in, so now it is up to you to draw on this money for as long as possible, so that the total amount you will receive from your Social Security, pension, and annuity will be as large as possible!

Money That Is Not Guaranteed, That You Can Outlive, but That You Can Also Pass On

In this second category is money you can outlive, that is not guaranteed, but which, if you do not spend it all before you die, can be passed on to your heirs, to your estate, or to charity. These monies or resources can include:

- Stocks and bonds not in a retirement account (qualified retirement accounts are subject to different rules than non-qualified accounts)
- Rental property income or royalty income
- Your principal residence

STOCKS AND BONDS NOT IN A
RETIREMENT ACCOUNT

On a day-to-day basis, it is wisest for you to spend only the money generated as interest and dividends on your holdings. It is important that you resist the urge to withdraw and/or liquidate your holdings for a perceived "emergency" or for "special occasions." It is imperative to understand that withdrawals and liquidations will reduce the critical mass of such accounts and thus reduce your ongoing income from these sources. This is clearly not a recommended strategy as it cannibalizes one's future retirement income.

RENTAL PROPERTY OR RENTAL INCOME, AND
ROYALTIES ON YOUR INTELLECTUAL PROPERTY

Similarly, it will be best to consume only the income generated from these resources. As with stocks and bonds, you can sell some of these income-producing properties for the special situation, but this will result in less money coming in on a regular basis. Accordingly, the watchword for the conscientious planner is preservation, not liquidation, of capital, for all the reasons discussed in the section on stocks and bonds.

YOUR PRINCIPAL RESIDENCE

There are several ways in which your principal residence can serve as a source of income. You can borrow against it. You can sell it and use the proceeds as additional income. In that regard, if you sell your home, just not paying the real estate taxes on your principal residence will probably pay for half the rent that you might need to pay after you've sold your house. However, it is best to recall that the cost of rent is related to market factors and can increase accordingly; today's savings are not guaranteed to continue when you rent property.

Yet another source of additional income to explore is the interesting world of reverse mortgages. If you own your home outright, which many retirees do, and if you do not plan to leave your home to one of your children or other relatives, this may well be a way of generating additional income. With a reverse mortgage, you essentially trade your home for a significant amount of income for as long as you live while continuing to live in your home. Thereafter the home belongs to the company selling you the reverse mortgage. There are many downsides to this type of transaction, and it is a transaction that is probably best not entered into unless there is a dire need for additional income on your part. If you must enter into a reverse mortgage, retain aggressive legal counsel prior to exploring the minefield of reverse mortgages.

New Money or Earned Income in Retirement

If you find that the income you currently receive in retirement is not sufficient for your needs, or that the income you expected to have has been seriously diminished by events like the Great Recession of 2008, you may have to develop additional sources of income. There are a number of ways you can do this. These include:

- Going back to work, full-time or part-time
- Consulting
- Starting your own business
- Investing
- Selling on eBay, or craigslist, or in consignment stores

Each of these options has certain advantages and disadvantages. Let's consider each of them in turn:

GOING BACK TO WORK, FULL-TIME OR PART-TIME

One option for earning additional income is to go back to work, either at your previous job or one similar to what you used to do. That way you do not have to acquire a whole new set of skills. You can do so part-time or full-time, as you wish and your financial needs dictate. Many people who have done so have been very satisfied with both the additional income and the meaningful social contact and interactions. Finding a job not in your area of expertise is usually less reward-ing financially, although it may have other benefits, such as learning about a whole new field, or meeting an entirely new set of people. Examples of such new activi-ties might be: selling real estate; working in retail sales; substitute teaching; neighborhood babysitting; or sub-stituting at the post office at Christmas time. Again, the possibilities are almost endless, since you are trying to earn only some additional income to *supplement* the re-tirement income you already have.

CONSULTING

If you have been successful in your profession, your business, or your trade, your accumulated wisdom and skills may well be marketable: you can become an ex-pert consultant on what you know or what you do well. Consulting can bring you many benefits. It can provide additional income and often a flexible schedule, one you can set for yourself. In addition, consulting may involve travel to interesting places. So, perhaps you might want to add a few vacation days to your consulting venue. You can let it be known informally to your previous work associates and friends that you are available as a consultant, or you could start your own Web site and advertise your services.

STARTING YOUR OWN BUSINESS

Another way that you could capitalize on your accumulated knowledge would be to start your own business, either in the field that you already know, or in a field that has been your avocation, but one in which you have acquired considerable knowledge and skill. You may have dreamed of opening your own restaurant, or a stamp collectors' shop, or a bike repair shop, or any one of a thousand ideas that may have come your way. Again, this could be a lot of fun, and it might provide additional income.

INVESTING

Another possibility is to try your hand at *investing*. Since investing does not guarantee that you will actually make money, you should do so only with money you can afford to lose; I call this your "play money." You can try your hand at investing in an industry or in a stock that you understand well and think has promise for the future. Or you can even try day-trading, if you can pay continuing attention to the market. If you are brand new to investing, it may be best to do so under the guidance of an experienced mentor whom you trust absolutely. A word of caution: while many people have realized tremendous gains derived from personally investing in the financial markets, it is also an unfortunate reality that many have lost money which they could not afford to lose by speculating in financial markets. Investments today are increasingly complex and subject to a myriad of geopolitical and economic influences. Accordingly, they may best be left in the hands of highly skilled and experienced analysts.

SELLING ON EBAY AND CRAIGSLIST AND IN CONSIGNMENT STORES

Over a lifetime, many of us have accumulated valuable "treasures" that we are probably not going to use any longer. You could have fun selling them for a little extra income. Such items might include jewelry, art, electronics, a second car that you don't need anymore, etc. You could have fun doing this yourself, since it doesn't take long to learn how to use eBay or craigslist. For example, Linda, a social worker, has been a life-long collector of dolls and certain Hallmark products. When she retired, she had a lot of fun, and made considerable profit, selling items in her collection on eBay. Or, if you do not wish to bother about selling items yourself, there are now businesses that will sell items on your behalf, for a modest commission. An additional benefit is that you will be able to unclutter your home, making it easier for you if you ever have to move again.

Three More Bits of Advice

There are three more bits of advice that I can give to assure that you have ample income in your retirement years:

- Work very hard, alone or with your financial advisor or tax accountant, to keep your income taxes as low as possible
- Avoid scams
- Consider getting a professional financial advisor

Keeping Your Income Tax as Low as Possible

Of course, you've probably pursued the goal of keeping your income taxes as low as possible throughout your lifetime. But it is particularly important to redouble your efforts in this regard in your later years. The tax system is constructed to seek to recoup taxes that were deferred during the working years. Thus, most so-called retirement income is subject to taxation, as is the majority of your Social Security income.

One specific strategy to pursue in this regard is to take advantage of any of the accrued and possibly deferred capital losses that you may have incurred during the 2008–2009 economic downturn. Not only can you deduct $3,000 of losses from your total income each year, but also any capital gains that you earn during the next few years can be offset by carry-over losses which many individuals have logged during the just-mentioned period.

Another strategy is to consider converting funds that have been accumulated in a traditional IRA to a Roth IRA. Then, if you are successful in making these funds grow in retirement, you will be able to draw on them tax-free. Also, if you are engaged in even a modest business enterprise, all of the expenses associated with conducting this business, as well as any losses incurred in running such a business, can be used to reduce your total tax liability.

One final strategy that you may wish to consider, especially if you are already inclined to make charitable contributions, is to consider arranging for a charitable gift annuity now. This will give you a large tax deduction in the year you arrange for such an annuity and a guaranteed income for you and your co-annuitant's lifetime. In addition, a sizeable proportion of the income derived from such an annuity will be tax exempt. It would be wise to ask various charitable organizations to whom you are considering leaving some of your money after you die to give you detailed illustrations of the specific costs and benefits involved in arranging for a charitable gift annuity. A brief illustration of some of the benefits of such an effort is detailed below. However, I strongly advise that you consider any and all of such tax-reduction strategies only with the full participation of a trusted tax advisor.

Larry Samson, age 73, attended an Ivy League school and now wants to establish a gift annuity at his alma mater to benefit needy students who could not otherwise afford to attend that school. He makes a donation of $100,000 to his former school. In return he will receive an annuity payout of $6,200 each year as long as he lives. In addition he will be able to take a $31,900 tax deduction in the year he makes the gift, and approximately $4,200 of his annual payout will be received tax free, with the remaining $2,000 being taxed at his ordinary income tax rate. Larry is so pleased with these results that in the next year he repeats the process, giving another $100,000 to his school, and receiving a similar tax deduction and similar annuity payouts. In addition, the president of the university invites Larry to a VIP reception honoring him and other major donors to the university. He meets classmates he has not seen for years and has a wonderful time reconnecting.

Looks like a win-win situation to me.

Avoid Scams

Beware! Older people are prime targets for scams, swindles, rip-off home repairs, Ponzi schemes, and a variety of other traps offered by opportunists. You must be vigilant to avoid falling prey to these criminals. Scams against the elderly can take many forms. Among the most common are unnecessary repairs, services offered by unlicensed or unqualified service providers, or service providers who ask to be paid for services before a service is rendered and who never deliver. You need to be very wary of people who come to your door saying they are working in the neighborhood and offering you a service, such as trimming your trees, fixing your roof, painting your house, or similar services. You are much better off seeking a service provider yourself, based on a solid recommendation from someone you know who has had a satisfactory experience with that service provider.

Virginia was an 87-year-old widow who lived alone in a pleasant residential neighborhood. A nice-looking young man knocked on her door, told her he was "working in the neighborhood," and that he noticed some missing shingles on her roof that he would be happy to repair at minimal cost. He offered to go onto the roof and inspect the damage in more detail. She invited him to do so, and he came back, looking very concerned, and said that he had discovered quite a few areas that needed to have shingles replaced. He offered to repair the damage for a mere $500 total, and in order for him to buy the appropriate supplies she would have to pay him $200 up front. He said she could pay him the rest of the money after he completed the work. She gave him the $200, and she is still waiting for his return. A neighbor who heard about this problem went up on her roof and found there was actually no damage to be fixed. He warned her not to fall prey again to service people who come knocking on her door.

Other scams sometimes perpetrated against the elderly are promises of high rates of interest or high rates of return on an "investment" from individuals or companies whose real intent is to defraud the elderly. Such companies may use the "investments" from new participants to initially pay high rates of return to the original investors, only to dissolve or disappear from the face of the earth once they have collected sufficient money from gullible investors. One bit of advice is that "if it sounds too good to be true, it probably is." The case of Bernie Madoff, who operated a successful Ponzi scheme for many years and stole billions of dollars from his victims, is only too well known. He was successful because he appeared to be such a trustworthy and knowledgeable person who was recommended by other satisfied clients. Too many individuals have been hurt by schemes like these. You must use an abundance of caution when responding to come-ons through the mail, by e-mail, in newspapers and magazines, or through unsolicited telephone calls. Beware!

Consider Getting a Financial Advisor

Just in case this all sounds too complicated for you, you can go a different route: Instead of making all these decisions yourself, you can employ a financial advisor. But you must apply considerable caution here as well. Many people offering financial advice do so by offering the services they sell. Brokers are compensated for their efforts on your behalf, and it is your responsibility to read all the disclosure materials provided by your broker and then make an informed decision.

CHAPTER SUMMARY

- Everything you want to do in retirement depends on an adequate stream of income, most important of which is an adequate amount of money that you and your partner cannot outlive.

- Have some additional monies that you can use for special occasions, to have fun, and—if the money outlasts you—that you can pass on to your heirs or to worthy causes.

- Be prepared to generate additional income, if needed, by continuing to work, consulting, or even starting a new business.

- Work toward keeping your taxes as low as possible.

- Beware of scams, opportunists, Ponzi schemes.

- Consider investing, but know what you are doing. Or get professional help from a financial advisor, but be careful as well in selecting a financial advisor.

- "And the money keeps rolling in." Strive to achieve and maintain *financial* fitness so you will be able to relax in financial security.

Chapter 10

Exercise Every Day, and Make It Fun

THIS CHAPTER discusses the unique role that exercise plays in maintaining wellness. If exercise were a pill, it would be the most prescribed medication throughout life and especially in retirement. The benefits of exercise are numerous, and they are enormous:

- Exercise will make you a better all-around person.
- Exercise will make you a happier person.
- Exercise will increase your sex appeal. (Who wouldn't want that?)
- Exercise will retard aging. Inactivity accelerates aging.

The goal of this chapter is not to simply advise you of the many benefits of regular, vigorous exercise but also to show you how you can implement this advice in your own life, regardless of what your exercise practice has been until now.

Exercise, while extremely valuable, can also be boring if you don't find ways to make it fun. So don't *just* exercise: Dance! Swim! Play! Play golf, play tennis, or walk, walk, walk instead! Make exercise a thoroughly enjoyable as well as a social activity, and integrate it fully into your lifestyle.

Whether we look at research or look at cultures in which nearly everyone lives to a ripe old age, exercise trumps virtually every other factor as a positive contributor to longevity. To achieve a long and active life, we need to maintain mobility and flexibility. Accordingly, my advice to you is to *exercise vigorously every day of your life.*

The Goals of Exercise

The goals of exercise are manifold: to retain mobility; to increase muscle tissue and muscle tone; to reduce body fat; to strengthen bones; to retain flexibility; to exercise the heart regularly; and to improve your mood. To meet these goals, we must make a commitment to vigorously exercise every day. Fortunately, there are many different ways in which to meet this goal, at any age, under any circumstances. Vigorous sports, dancing, brisk walking, and the use of a stationary or a recumbent bicycle or exercise machines are available and affordable. You can overcome bad weather by exercising inside your home or by going to the mall for a vigorous walk. Gyms are almost universally available and fairly affordable. You can exercise alone, with a partner, or with friends.

The two most beneficial types of exercise are (1) cardiovascular exercise, which involves rapid activity that increases the heart rate, such as in running, dancing, swimming, or bicycling; and (2) muscle-building activity, such as lifting weights or exercising against mechanical resistance. These two types are complementary. Exercising with weights, or exertion against resistance, builds one's store of muscle, which then acts as a basic "bank account" for a healthy life. Cardiovascular exercise improves cardiac capacity and circulation. Both kinds are needed and indicated.

Types of Exercise

Walking Briskly

Walking briskly is probably the easiest form of exercise to accomplish. It can get you out in nature. It requires virtually no equipment except a good pair of walking shoes and comfortably fitting clothing. It can be done nearly everywhere, alone or with others, while working or playing. Ten thousand steps a day is a reasonable goal. I recommend that you get a pedometer that keeps track of all your steps during planned exercise as well as during your routine daily activities. This is a relatively small investment to make. Recently, a number of organizations, such as AARP, have been giving away pedometers when you sign up for membership, but you can also purchase one at your local drug store.

Stationary Bikes and Other Exercise Machines

If any limitation, such as arthritis, back problems, or other physical impediment, prevents you from walking briskly on a regular basis, use a stationary bike every day. Upright or recumbent bikes provide you with a very good form of cardiovascular exercise. Other exercise machines to consider are elliptical trainers, treadmills, and StairMasters. Most such machines are equipped with measuring instruments that allow you to see how many minutes, miles, or calories you have achieved with the exercise. An additional advantage of such bikes is they hardly ever wear out. And, you can also do other things while exercising on a stationary or a recumbent bike or other exercise machines, such as watching television or reading a magazine or a book.

Add Strength Training to Cardiovascular Exercise

You need some kind of strength training to help you build muscle mass, especially in your arms, your upper body, and your back. An increase in muscle mass increases your basic metabolic rate and is especially effective in reducing abdominal fat deposits. Strength training will require a set of free weights or dumb-bells, or elastic resistance bands designed for strength training. Or you may make use of strength-training equipment in a gym. If you decide to use such equipment, it is best to get instruction from a professional trainer to get you started so that you will learn proper technique and avoid any injury. Strength training is also important from an aesthetic point of view as it can help to reshape your body into more attractive proportions.

Chart Your Progress

Charting your exercise progress is useful because it provides you with accountability. Both cardiovascular exercise and strength-building exercise should be performed incrementally until you have achieved your desired goals and your exercise pattern has become a well-established habit. At that point it may no longer be necessary to keep charts, but it may still be useful to keep a running log of your activities to keep you accountable and to avoid any slippage in your exercise pattern.

Restart Exercise Activities after Any Period of Forced Inactivity

If your exercise routine is interrupted by hospitalization, an injury, or an acute illness, you need to restart your exercise program as soon as possible. Muscles start to atrophy very quickly with inactivity, and you will also lose flexibility. Accordingly, you need to gradually resume exercising until you work back up to your former high level of activity. Remember, all the benefits listed at the beginning of this chapter will accrue to you when you get "back in form." You'll once again look better, feel better, and accomplish more!

Overcome Obstacles to Exercising Regularly

Many of the obstacles we encounter in our efforts to exercise regularly no longer exist once you have retired. The old excuses that you just don't have time or that you are too busy just don't wash anymore. You are in charge of your own schedule now. The fact that you are out of shape is also no longer a barrier to exercising, since you can start slowly and increase your activities gradually. In addition, here is a little secret: regular exercise generates pleasure hormones that will make you enjoy exercise a lot more. Yes, you are literally becoming addicted—to exercise.

Make Exercise a Social Occasion

In retirement you will find many other people in your neighborhood, your church, synagogue, or other social groups who also need to exercise. Join them, or invite them to exercise with you. One of the pleasures of exercising with others is that this brings many other rewards: contact, connectedness, and sociability. You will find that you look forward to talking as well as exercising with these companions. In addition, you can take pride in the fact that you are contributing to others' well-being and enjoyment of life. And, you may find that you have other things in common with your walking partners, and this may lead to additional joint activities. Or, if you need further incentives, consider getting a dog that needs and enjoys walking. Having a dog brings other rewards as well; you can start up a conversation in your neighborhood around your dog, or you can share what you have in common with other people walking their dogs. So, little by little, there are *no more excuses* and *a lot more incentives.* So, move!

Consider Working with a Personal Trainer

If you are unable to motivate yourself to get into a pattern of regular, vigorous, muscle-building activity, consider working with a personal trainer. I have seen the most dramatic results—almost total transformation of the body—when people who needed to exercise and couldn't bring themselves to stick with a program finally sought the services of a personal trainer. A personal trainer teaches, motivates, and rewards you. Do it, if that is what it takes. Here is an example of how this can work:

Dr. A. was a very well-respected internist in his mid-50s. He was moderately successful in his practice, but he craved to crank it up another notch. One thing that was holding him back was that he was some 50 pounds over-weight. When he admonished his diabetic or hypertensive patients who had gained too much weight, he wasn't very convincing. He had tried dieting many times, each time losing a few pounds, only to gain them back rapidly. He was frustrated. So he decided to try a new approach. He hired a personal trainer.

Within three months he had accomplished what he hadn't been able to accomplish in ten years. He lost 40 pounds, acquired a new wardrobe, and enjoyed a whole new outlook on life. He became so revitalized that he decided to open a new kind of practice: concierge medicine for a somewhat smaller number of patients with whom he emphasized preventive medicine practices. The difference was that now he could hold himself out as an example for his patients to follow. He continued to treat a few of his established patients who wanted this kind of special service, and he recruited quite a few new patients. After not having seen him for several months, I ran into him at a social occasion. He looked great, and I told him so. He beamed and said to me simply: "I got a personal trainer."

Become Passionate about Exercise

The best way to assure that you will always reap all the benefits that exercise has to offer is to become passionate about exercise. Relish seeing your body in motion and seeing it gain strength, flexibility, and endurance. Get excited over the fact that you can initiate this wonderful activity at will, and that you can do so every day. Passion and fatigue are incompatible with one another, and regardless of how "tired" you may feel from your other activities, demands, and chores, exercise will abolish this so-called fatigue, until, after an extended period of time, it is replaced with well-earned *physical* fatigue for which rest, and eventually sleep, will become a great restorer. In fact, passion about exercise is necessary in order for you to attain the sense of well-being and control that only regular vigorous physical activity can provide. It will then allow you to become, or to remain, passionate about all of your other life goals and endeavors. And passion is the engine required to achieve every goal.

Harvest the Health Benefits of Your Exercise Program

I recommend that you work closely with your doctor to harvest all the health benefits of your successful exercise program. Did you know that you might be able to reduce the amount and number of medications you take if you have any of the following chronic diseases: diabetes, hypertension, cardiovascular disease, and even osteoporosis? All of these will benefit from the work of the twin engines of your exercise program: cardiovascular exercise and strength training. Your exercise program will also reduce your risk of falling and its resulting injuries.

Exercise, and Make It Fun

No matter how persuasive all the information about the benefits of exercise is, you may not be able to stick with it unless you also make exercise fun. There are a number of ways you can do this. Regular vigorous exercise in itself produces pleasure-producing hormones that make regular exercise virtually addictive—a good kind of addiction, if I may say so. But there are also other ways of assuring that exercise is fun. One way is to reward yourself every time you achieve one of your exercise goals. What kinds of rewards will work for you? Perhaps a new wardrobe? Or going on a mini-vacation? Or, maybe praise from yourself or from someone you care about is enough. Mutual praise is a great reward system, and yet another reason to exercise with someone else. Here is another illustration of what exercise can do:

> Ralph and Sharon were far too busy during their working years, he as an architect and she as a nurse, to spend much time thinking about exercise. They were naturally slim and had never been overweight. Neither were they ever particularly athletic. However, when their careers ended, and they had little to do other than maintaining their small home and yard, they decided to become serious walkers. Each morning and evening, for the past 10 years, they have been walking together through their neighborhood. Sometimes they must dress warmly against the cold, and sometimes they walk only very early in the day and late at night to avoid the summertime heat. It has brought them closer together. Ralph now has a heart condition that limits his exercise tolerance, so they walk at a slower pace than they used to, but they still walk, often hand in hand, and

often stopping to talk to their neighbors, sharing news and information. Everyone knows Ralph and Sharon and feels close to them. Now in their early 80s, they plan to continue their walking journey for many more years to come, if possible. They are convinced that exercise retards aging and that inactivity accelerates aging.

CHAPTER SUMMARY

- Exercise! Exercise every day!
- Don't just exercise—Dance! Swim! Play!
- Exercise will make you a better all-around person.
- Exercise will make you a happier person.
- Exercise will increase your sex appeal.
- Incorporate exercise into your lifestyle.
- Emphasize cardiovascular training.
- Add strength training to cardiovascular exercise.
- Become passionate about exercise.
- Consider getting a personal trainer.
- Make exercise a social occasion.
- Harvest the health benefits of your successful exercise program.
- So, exercise, and make it fun!

Chapter 11

Protect Your
Independence

I N THIS CHAPTER I discuss strategies for maintaining your independence and for avoiding dependency. It's worth fighting for your independence. Moreover, it is much easier to maintain
independence than to regain it. And any episode of dependency should be regarded as strictly temporary, to
be reversed as soon as possible. Dependency, especially
when there is reduced mobility on the part of the patient or when the patient is bedridden, brings with it a
meltdown of bone and muscle within weeks, and it can
lead to other serious health problems, such as pressure
ulcers and bone demineralization. These complications
of even temporary dependency are to be avoided at all
costs. At the same time, it is wise to prepare for a time
when dependency cannot be avoided altogether. And it

will be much easier to accept dependency if you have someone on whom you can actually depend, that is, someone to assist you with activities you can no longer perform yourself. It also helps if that person is someone whom you trust absolutely. Accordingly, I recommend some advance planning for such a possibility as you grow older. It's a good idea to evaluate available in-home and facility-based caregivers, though home is clearly the best option, or at least as "home-like" as is possible. This chapter offers strategies for maintaining functional independence and avoiding physical dependency. The following story illustrates that independence is worth fighting for:

> Albert was a retired electrical engineer who had worked for a regional telephone company for more than 30 years. One of the jobs he worked on for the company was designing and installing the 911 emergency call system in his community. After he retired he used his considerable skills to carry out a number of home improvement projects, including building a workshop for his woodworking activities, enclosing a carport, and making some cabinet repairs in his kitchen. He also made himself available for similar repair tasks at the church that he attended, and he car-

ried out a number of complex handyman tasks at the homes of friends. It was clear that he had valuable skills, that he enjoyed using those skills, and that he relished the appreciation his various repair projects earned him.

One afternoon, after he had just finished replacing a faucet in his kitchen, he suddenly fell over onto the hallway floor and was unable to get up. His speech was slurred, and although he tried to get up, he could not and repeatedly fell back to the floor. His wife quickly recognized that he had probably suffered a major stroke. She immediately called 911 (the very system that Albert had designed and helped install), and an ambulance arrived in short order. The medics took him to the local general hospital's emergency room. He was quickly seen by a neurologist and had a CAT scan of his brain done which confirmed that he had had a stroke but that there was no brain hemorrhage. He was treated with a clot-dissolving medication and admitted to the hospital.

The next day his speech returned partially, and he was able to move his right leg a little when asked to do so. After several days of in-bed physical therapy he was admitted to the rehabilitation section of the hospital and advised that he would need several weeks of intense physical therapy to retrain his muscles and brain. He was also started on daily speech therapy to recover his ability to communicate clearly. As was his style, Albert participated vigorously in his rehabilitation activities. And with the strong emotional support of his wife, his daughter, and several members of his congregation, he fully recovered the use of his leg and his speech. A test of his memory capacity three months after the initial episode showed that his memory, too, was functioning normally.

Months later still, after a leisurely vacation on one of Florida's beaches, he was back to looking for and completing fix-up projects in his own home and in a friend's house. His mood was good, and he felt he had dodged a bullet. There were no residual deficits as he cheerfully cut the birthday cake at the celebration of his 85th birthday. Both he and his wife, as well as his friends, knew that the outcome could have been so much worse.

What You Can Do to Avoid Dependency

Previous chapters have provided you with tools that are important for maintaining your independence: Chapter 6 covered the importance of and the strategies for maintaining your physical health—for example, you should treat any acute illness completely until you have fully recovered, and you should manage any chronic illness aggressively to assure that maximum rehabilitation is achieved and that the residual loss of functioning is minimized. Chapter 7 discussed maintaining your mental health, and Chapter 8 covered how to maintain your brain to keep your memory sharp. Chapter 10 stressed the importance of vigorous exercise in maintaining your well-being, while Chapters 3 and 5 dealt with the importance of choosing an ideal place to live and how to maintain your social connections. All of these topics contribute to your ability to maintain your physical, social, and financial independence. This chapter focuses on some other steps you need to take and additional issues you need to be aware of in order to retain your independence as you progress further into this phase of your life.

Stop Risk-Taking

It is now time to start "acting your age" and, as noted earlier, to avoid taking unnecessary risks. Do not climb ladders, do not walk on your roof to clean the gutters, do not learn to ski, and do not show off. Any fall and any broken bones that might result from such risk-taking behavior can lead to major damage and limitations that are simply not worth the benefits you might get from still carrying out such activities.

Fall-Proof Your Home

Before you need them, have grab-bars installed in your bathroom. Get rid of all throw rugs that you might slip and fall over. Put nightlights in your hallways and bathrooms. Don't rearrange your furniture too often, since you might not remember the changes when you walk about the house at night. Install railings on your front steps, and use the railings when going up a set of stairs, or when boarding an airplane, for instance. Your bones are thinner now and can break more easily.

Prepare for When You Are No Longer Totally Independent

Remember that you also need to prepare for a time when you are no longer totally independent. This may come about as a result of relatively minor conditions, such as arthritis, or as a result of increasing frailty with advancing age. During this phase of retirement you should arrange for alternate ways of performing some of the activities that you can no longer perform with ease, while maintaining a general sense of independent functioning. The important thing at this stage is to *maintain a sense of independence, even when you have become somewhat dependent.*

When to Stop Driving

Driving an automobile is an essential component of your independence. But eventually you will have to decide when to stop driving. This could come after you've had your first fender-bender, caused by inattention, or after you've had a heart attack or a stroke. Or, you could decide to stop driving before you are forced to do so, and you could *become chauffeur-driven.* This might be one of the wisest and most powerful decisions you can make: to stop driving *before* you have an accident that could injure yourself or someone else, to say nothing of the financial cost that such an accident might produce.

But you still have to have reliable transportation. Accordingly, you need to take time to think this through so that you have transportation available whenever you want it or need it. You actually have a number of choices: if you live in a city, taxis are probably your best bet. And the money you save on gasoline and car insurance could easily go into a "taxi fund." But if you don't live in a city, taxis aren't usually an option. If your partner can still drive, that's a great solution. If not, perhaps you'll need to find a volunteer from your church or congregation who is willing to take you places, or you'll need to hire someone who can drive you wherever you need to go.

Many retirement communities provide transportation for their residents for going to the mall, to the doctor, or for grocery shopping. Others have a group of volunteer drivers available. In certain communities, such as in Sun City Center, near Tampa, Florida, or in the Villages in central Florida, golf cart transportation is available when automobile travel is no longer feasible or advisable. The slower speeds of golf carts and golf cart travel lanes in such communities allow some people to extend their mobility when they no longer can or wish to drive. The bottom line is that you need to figure out how you are going to get where you want to go after giving up driving your own beloved automobile.

Maintain Your Financial Independence

While it is important to maintain physical independence, it is equally important to maintain financial independence. When you get to the point where it is difficult for you to write a check, or when you begin to have difficulty remembering when a payment is due, it will be best for you to have someone who can do this for you, either on a regular basis or whenever you need help. Having a joint checking account with your spouse or partner or an adult child can accomplish this. Or, you may need to give power of attorney to someone you trust, so that this person can initiate financial transactions at your request or on your behalf.

Consider Getting an Elder Law Attorney

An elder law attorney is someone who specializes in legal and financial issues related to people in retirement. Such an attorney can prepare appropriate legal documents for you, such as a power of attorney, a living will, advance directives, medical surrogate documents, a will, and a living trust. He or she may also be able to advise you on requirements for Medicaid eligibility, tax issues, and other late-in-life matters.

What to Do When You Become Dependent

Should you become physically dependent, it is most important to have someone you can depend on who can assist you with those activities that you yourself can no longer carry out. It is equally important that you continue to do all those things you can still do for yourself. Obviously this caregiver needs to be someone you can trust completely, who can make decisions on your behalf if you are no longer able to do so.

Things to Consider When Choosing Dependent-Care Providers

If or when you or your partner requires long-term dependent care, there are a number of issues to consider. These issues are similar whether the care is to be provided within your own home or in a long-term care facility. Foremost among these are the *comfort* and the *safety* of the person for whom care is provided. In terms of comfort, if at all possible, such care should be provided in the person's own home, or in a setting that is as "home-like" as possible. In terms of safety, the medical competency and the accreditation of the caregiver or the facility must be assured.

If you are looking for an in-home caregiver for your dependent loved one, it may be best to go through an accredited home health care agency of the local Visiting Nurse Association. You should personally interview the caregiver candidate to assure that he or she is going to be compatible with both you and the person for whom you are arranging care. You also want to make sure that the caregiver has sufficient experience with the kind of medical problem for which their help is sought.

Sometimes the best way of "lucking into" such a person is to hire someone who has recently finished caregiving for someone you know well who is no longer in need of such care. That way you will have a "user-proven" caregiver working with your loved one. In-home care can be provided by a person who comes into the home on a daily basis or by someone who is willing and able to be a live-in caregiver. The latter assumes that you have the capacity to provide live-in space for the caregiver. If you are looking for a facility to provide care for your dependent loved one, you should do similar "due diligence" in qualifying the facility. Visit the facility and speak with administrative as well as hands-on personnel. If at all possible, you should discuss the adequacy of such a facility with other persons who have had family members receive care there. Then you should plan to visit your loved one at the facility on a regular basis to assure that the kind of care you would expect is in fact being delivered. If it is not, you will need to discuss your concerns with the appropriate administrative and clinical personnel. If dissatisfactions can't be resolved in this way, you should search for an alternate facility.

Understand Long-Term Care

It is important for you to understand how long-term care is provided. I would have titled this section "Understanding the Long-term Care System," but unfortunately there is no actual *system* of long-term care in the United States. What does exist is a series of quasi-residential, quasi-medical facilities that provide some of the care that may be needed. Here is a brief guide to the kinds of facilities that provide long-term care:

ASSISTED LIVING FACILITIES

Assisted Living Facilities, or ALFs, are residential facilities that provide basic food and shelter for people who are no longer able to provide these for themselves. Medicare and Medicaid do not cover care in ALFs, but some long-term care insurance policies do. Some ALFs provide assistance only with basic self-care, while others may additionally provide medication administration and medical monitoring, such as blood pressure measurements or blood sugar testing.

REHABILITATION CENTERS

Rehabilitation centers are facilities that provide residential care plus rehabilitation activities such as physical therapy, occupational therapy, and speech therapy immediately following a hospitalization stay for a hip fracture or a stroke, for example. Medicare covers rehabilitation care for a specified period of time during which restorative care is medically necessary.

NURSING HOMES

Nursing homes provide care for individuals who are no longer able to care for themselves, either post-hospital or after an illness at home. They provide assistance with self-care, medication administration, and some medical services, such as nursing care. Many nursing homes are also staffed with social workers. Nursing homes operate under the supervision of a medical director, who must be a physician. The patient's personal physician, or the nurse practitioner or physician's assistant associated with that doctor, provides personal medical care. Most people would like to avoid care in a nursing home. However, when multiple types of care are needed that cannot be provided in the person's home, a nursing home is indeed the appropriate place to receive care.

Who Pays for Long-Term Care?

People often assume that Medicare covers the cost of long-term care. This is not the case. Medicare will cover only the cost of a limited number of days of rehabilitation if that episode of rehabilitation immediately follows hospital care. Medicaid covers the cost of long-term care only for individuals without financial resources or those who have "spent down" their resources to a minimum amount of income. A person may still own their own home and receive Medicaid benefits, but other types of financial resources must first be spent on the patient's care before Medicaid takes over. However, every state has its own rules for Medicaid eligibility. So who pays for long-term care if Medicaid does not? You do, unless you acquire long-term care insurance.

LONG-TERM CARE INSURANCE

This type of insurance provides for the cost of receiving long-term care for a chronic illness. Depending on the specific terms of your long-term care insurance policy, this can include the cost of a nursing home, an assisted living facility, or medical care that you receive in your home. The reason for insuring against long-term care costs is that these can be very high indeed, and they may continue over a period of months or even years. The cost of nursing home care may range anywhere from $60,000 to $120,000 per year, depending on where you live, with highest costs being in the Northeast and California and the lowest cost in southern states. Thus, over a period of several years, the cost of nursing home care can completely wipe out a considerable fortune.

The cost of long-term care insurance can be very reasonable and affordable if it is purchased for an individual who is still relatively healthy. The cost for such insurance for someone who already has a condition which is likely to result in long-term care, such as diabetes with complications or Alzheimer's disease, is almost prohibitively expensive and often not much less than the cost of paying for such care out of pocket. So it would be wise to acquire this type of insurance when the person to be covered is still free of any serious chronic disease. Also, be diligent in learning exactly what kind of services are covered by any long-term care insurance program offered to you.

CHAPTER SUMMARY

- Fight for your independence.
- Maintain physical independence.
- Know what you can do to avoid dependency.
- Stop risk-taking.
- Accident-proof your home.
- Prepare for when you are no longer totally independent.
- Know when to stop driving.
- Maintain financial independence.
- Consider working with an elder law attorney.
- Be ready for when dependence comes.
- Find someone on whom you can depend if you are going to be dependent.
- Understand who pays for long-term care.
- Consider acquiring long-term care insurance.

Chapter 12

Embrace Your Inner, Spiritual Self

WHEN WE think of people's inner lives—their dreams, fantasies, and a vivid imagination—we often think of this as being the province of the young. Thus far, relatively few authors have written about the inner lives of people in retirement. But recent research, including my own, has shown that individuals approaching retirement or in retirement *continue* to have a lively imagination and a rich inner world of dreams and fantasies.

In this chapter I encourage you to explore and cherish *your* inner life. It can actually be a source of great satisfaction and wonder to you, as it is one of the richest theaters of human experience yet discovered. I describe how you might best access your own inner life, and how to share it with others. Before discussing my own work on the inner life of the older person, I pay tribute to two distinguished colleagues who opened up this field of inquiry: psychiatrist Jack Weinberg, M.D., and psychologist James Birren, Ph.D. Weinberg, through psychoanalytic studies, and Birren, through guided autobiographical studies, have illuminated this field for me and others, and have whetted my appetite to pursue these studies further, and for this I am deeply grateful.

My own knowledge of the inner life of the older person stems largely from intensive clinical work with patients, supplemented by informal explorations with relatives, acquaintances, and friends. I have also learned a great deal about the inner life of older persons through teaching several courses in guided autobiography. I have gleaned nuggets of insight from interactions with deeply demented patients suffering from Alzheimer's disease. Some of these individuals, despite severe memory impairment, have at times offered surprising, poetic, and altogether astonishing insights into their minds. To all these individuals I am also extremely grateful.

My own interest in studying the inner life of people in their later years arose from the belief that something that was so important in younger years couldn't just disappear in later life. I found that if one looked for it, there emerged a rich and varied inner life that had not previously been studied or appreciated. In fact, what emerged was a picture of a noisy, lusty, dramatic, colorful, poetic, artistic, and always deeply moving inner experience well worth exploring and appreciating.

In order for you to explore your own inner life, either with a trusted friend or a trained counselor, a number of conditions must be present. Your friend or counselor must possess the following characteristics: an eager curiosity, a spontaneous response to your revelations, and an unconditional acceptance of both you and your revelations.

Techniques for Connecting with Your Inner Life

There are a number of specific techniques that have been found useful for accessing your own inner life. These include participating in guided reminiscences, or in a full-scale life review, with an experienced counselor; a personal examination of your lifetime goals;

writing your autobiography; exploring "dream jobs" you aspired to during your working years; exploring what you wanted to become as an adolescent; or exploring what kind of a person you always wanted to become in your retirement years. Another interesting approach I have used is to ask, "If you could be any kind of an animal, what kind of an animal would you like to be?" Or, somewhat irreverently, I like to ask the elderly, "Who do you want to be when you grow up?" As you can see, a certain degree of playfulness is involved in this approach to a person's fantasy life. So here are a few illustrations of how this works:

Dream Jobs. Joffre Dumazedier, a French sociologist, found that the majority of individuals in the workforce have, in addition to the job they actually hold, a fantasy or dream job that they would rather do than the one they actually have. Thus, a university president might wish to be the captain of a pleasure boat; a chief financial officer might wish to be a social worker; a biochemist might wish to lead a Boy Scout troop; a psychiatrist might wish to be a bartender, and so on. Exploring your fantasies about your dream jobs can tell you a great deal about your inner life. It can even be a guide to the kind of activity you might still wish to undertake in retirement.

Adolescent Identities. Most individuals can recall some of their trial identities from their adolescence. These, too, can be quite revealing, since some of them may still be current aspirations or fantasies that have been too long suppressed. In fact, most adolescents toyed with many trial identities before they settled into the one identity that eventually shaped their lives. These explorations are not forgotten and may still be meaningful as you contemplate all that you may still wish to do. So, for instance, my trial identities included being a gardener, an actor, a politician, a writer, and a world traveler. What were yours? You may be surprised at what you once thought of doing or becoming. And there may be some things you might still give a try now that you are retired.

What Kind of Animal Would You Like to Be? This is perhaps the most interesting of the techniques for getting a glimpse into the inner life of a person. It cuts through a lot of resistance by making a game out of it. And it cuts directly to *images* in the inner life of that person. Most people find it easy to name an animal that they would like to be. Try it, and then go on to explore the qualities and characteristics of the animal that you might like to be.

Results of Such Explorations

The first and perhaps the most important finding from these explorations is that in their retirement years many people still experience a rich and varied inner life that is often directly or indirectly related to their self-esteem, their life satisfaction, and their self-image.

The second most interesting result is that the dominant mode that the inner life takes is the *visual mode;* that is, *images rather than ideas,* pop up. Furthermore, these images tend to *pull or draw* the individual's behavior in the direction of those images.

The third most interesting finding is that the nature of the themes and images which emerge from these explorations, is, perhaps not surprisingly, quite different for men and for women. Among women, generally, the dominant themes are for *freedom* and for *adulation.* One woman may describe herself as wanting to be "a bird, winging free, going where it wants to, without fetters or obligations." Or another woman may want to be "a cat, that comes and goes as it pleases, admired by everyone, but just walking away when she has had enough." These explorations and images hint at strong resentments over past repressions, past burdens, life-long obligations. They veritably scream, "Enough! I've given all my life. When do I get mine?" Again, these images may vividly illuminate what is not yet perfect in the person's life and may lead to activities which generate a better match between what is and what could be.

Interestingly, among most men a different set of themes surfaces: a longing for a childhood home, absolute security, abundant love, a return to their mother, or, at times, having great power over others. "I see myself walking across the old farm back in Alabama; my mother is calling for me," one man dreams. Another man sees himself as a foal, asleep in the warmth and safety of a country barn. Yet another man pictures himself as a hawk swooping down and gazing at all that is below him.

What becomes clear is that there is often a considerable distance between what people are and what they would like to be. And this is the exciting part: there is a chance in retirement to become or do anything that one may still want to become or do (see discussion in Chapter 4).

On a more philosophical basis, we may then also speculate whether similar themes emerge among future generations or among differing cultures. What I have discussed here applies largely to people in the United States, at this time in our history, among middle and upper-middle class individuals.

Your Spiritual Self

We are *spiritual* as well as physical beings. Most people, when they think of spirituality, think of religion. This usually means participating in a formal religious group. Religious belief and religious practices include a conceptual view of the world and each individual in it.

There are many religions, with many denominations, each with a somewhat unique set of tenets and assumptions. Most religions spell out what constitutes proper conduct in human life, and how the individual relates to a higher form of being, conceptualized as God, Allah, Yahweh, etc. The poet-philosopher Hafiz (who himself was described as the poet of the invisible) described this variety as "the different names of the one God."

Religions are meant to nourish the human spirit, to help us understand the complexity of the world we live in, and to adjust to good fortune as well as adversity. Because people vary widely, differing religions serve the needs of different people. While the majority of people are "brought up" in the religion of their parents, there is room for changing religious belief systems and religious affiliations as people mature. What is common to most religions is that they strongly support individual members, and that they constitute a strong community within the larger society. So strong is that sense of community that members of many religions refer to each other as "brother" and "sister."

Deep respect should be accorded to all varieties of religious belief. At the same time it is true that throughout history, and still to the present time, differing belief systems have at times been the source of hostility and conflict. Wars have been and are still being fought in the name of specific religions, supporting the believers and attacking the infidels. But it would be best to respect all religious systems as helpful to the people who subscribe to them. In general, religions promote altruism, kindness, and benevolence toward other human beings.

The Practical Value of Religious Practice

The principal benefit of belonging to a religious community is in quality of life. But a number of *practical* benefits also accrue to those involved in a religious congregation. Members of a congregation support one another in times of illness or economic distress. The social supports that flow to members of such a community can facilitate recovery from illness and help to overcome life's adversities. Beyond this, there is some research evidence that people with strong religious or other spiritual belief systems have stronger immune systems that help resist disease. Prayer, meditation, and yoga practice have all been shown in some studies to improve survival from major illnesses. Even if benefits cannot be universally demonstrated, no one has ever shown any negative effects from these activities. An exception may be the "true believer" who refuses needed medical care for himself or for a member of his family. In some such instances the courts have overruled those who refuse needed medical care for their children.

Non-Religious Forms of Spirituality

What has just been said about religious forms of spirituality applies equally well to non-religious forms of spirituality. There are systems of spirituality that do not postulate a specific religious belief system or a named superior being or spirit. These systems of spirituality are nevertheless powerful and meaningful to those adhering to them. Examples of such systems might be rational humanism or naturalism. To some extent, even atheism can be described as a kind of "religion."

These systems of spirituality extol the special humanity of each individual, and emphasize qualities of being that are other than physical or material. Both religious and non-religious forms of spirituality postulate the concept of a soul. The soul is more than the mind and the body. It is neither rational nor irrational. It simply *is*. According to most belief systems, the soul is what makes us human. It is what distinguishes us from other living things. It is what gives meaning to our lives. It is what pushes us to make an art of life. It lets us hear the sound of the trees when no wind stirs. It is our source of deep, imperturbable peace. It may be impossible to define the word *soul* precisely, but it has to do with genuineness and depth. It allows us to experience everyday things with intense awareness.

Another way to think of spirituality is to say that it is the opposite of materialism and consumerism. Being in touch with one's soul is what the poet Wallace Stevens said was "finding what will suffice." It allows us to live in a harmonious relationship with all of nature and all the creatures in it, including all of humanity.

The concept of a *soul mate* is interesting in this regard. It is used most commonly to define an ideal romantic relationship. But it derives from the idea of a unique individuality that can perhaps be matched by the unique individuality of another person.

I also need to point out that the word *psyche,* as the root word in *psychiatry* and *psychology,* refers to the care or the treatment of the soul. Today, however, we define psychiatrists and psychologists as experts on the mind and as healers of mental illness (as discussed in Chapter 7). For our purposes here, however, I refer to spirituality, or the soul, as what makes us uniquely human. It is important to acknowledge the existence of spirituality in yourself and in other people, and to know that care of the soul never ends.

Chapter Summary

- Realize you have a rich inner life.
- Access your inner life.
- Relish your inner life.
- Use your inner life as your guide.
- Realize you are also a spiritual being.
- Realize that there are many ways to be spiritual.
- One way of being spiritual is through membership in a formal religion.
- Other forms of spirituality exist outside of formal religions.
- The concept of a soul exists in both religious and non-religious forms of spirituality.
- The soul is neither rational nor irrational. It cannot be defined precisely.
- The soul allows us to live with intense awareness of ordinary things in our lives, and to make an art of life.
- Spirituality transcends the physical and the material world.
- Care of the soul never ends.

Chapter 13

Maintain Your Sexual Life

THIS CHAPTER addresses an often-overlooked aspect of aging: continued sexuality. My own research, and that of others, indicates that the vast majority of older people are interested in continuing their sex lives, even though the expression of sexuality may change somewhat in the later years.

Is Sexuality Still a Taboo Subject?

Believe me, despite the so-called "sexual revolution" of the 1960s, sexuality continues to remain a somewhat taboo subject, *especially for doctors.* The reason I share this somewhat shameful secret with you is that you may encounter such an attitude in *your* doctor, if and when you bring up the topic of sex with him or her. I can bet you dollars to doughnuts that your doctor *will not be the one to bring up the subject.* Many doctors shy away from discussing sexuality in older men and women because it seems to them like discussing the sex lives of their own mother or father. But more significantly, your doctor, unless he or she is exceptional, may not have a lot of information to offer you. Time and time again, my older patients have told me that when they brought up the subject, their doctor became uncomfortable and moved on to another subject. So you may have an opportunity to educate your doctors about sex among older people: to let them know, if this is true for you, that you are still interested in sex and what adjustments you have to make to be able to continue an active sex life. In truth, sex still seems to be considered a prerogative of the young in many quarters. But you and I know better.

I began my own research on sex in older people when I was still a medical student at Washington University in St. Louis, and I later continued these studies at the Duke University Center on Aging. I was fascinated that in the Duke University Longitudinal Study on Aging, the study pioneered by my mentor Ewald Busse, actually included questions about sexual behavior. However, the young doctors employed to collect this information often skipped asking the question about sexuality of their elderly subjects. Nonetheless, I found that the considerable amount of data that was accumulated in the data files of this study had never been analyzed by anyone. This gave me an immediate access to data that had been collected but ignored.

So I began to analyze and publish the data from this study. The results were really quite amazing. Yes, older people were still *interested* in sex, into their 60s, 70s, and occasionally even into their 80s. However, actual sexual activity began to decline in the 70s and beyond, more so among women than men. The reason? Women in their 70s were much less likely to have sexually active partners, as sexual activity dropped somewhat among men in their 70s. More importantly, however, many of the women in their 70s were widowed, and therefore no longer had an available sexual partner. Women were reluctant to establish new sexual relationships when they were in their 70s. Even if they wanted to, fewer and fewer unattached men were available. This is in part due to the fact that men on average die four years earlier than women, and the men had married women three years younger than they were. These women were essentially destined to live in widowhood for an average of seven years. That is the simple math that determines sexual expression in older women. While these studies were done in the 1950s and 1960s, the facts as they relate to sex in old age have not changed all that much. So what are the facts currently?

Men Continue to Be Interested in Sex into Their 70s

Men continue to be interested in sex well into their 70s, but their actual participation in sex declines markedly during this period. This is due to a number of factors: the accumulation of disabling chronic illnesses, for one, and lowered level of the male sex hormone, testosterone, for another. Plus, men in this age group experience a declining ability to have and maintain satisfactory erections. Erectile dysfunction occurs with a number of illnesses, especially diabetes. It can also occur as a side effect of medications the men may be taking, such as antihypertensive and antidepressant medications, as well as medications prescribed for prostatic hypertrophy. A variety of medications can also suppress sexual desire. So that's just how things were until relatively recently.

Along Came Viagra

Viagra became available for the first time in 1998. Here is one instance where scientific advances, combined with good old American commercialism, have brought about significant changes. You can't watch more than an hour of television without being bombarded with advertisements for drugs for what is now called E.D., short for erectile dysfunction, perhaps a more acceptable term for what used to be called impotence. Viagra has been highly successful, both scientifically and commercially, and has drawn other competitors for the treatment of erectile dysfunction. The "little blue pill" works, and it has changed the landscape, as it relates to sexuality, significantly. It has also given doctors at least one thing they can do for patients with erectile dysfunction. The availability of drugs for the treatment of erectile dysfunction has brought with it other changes in attitude and behavior, for example, greater willingness to discuss sexual matters in aging persons. And why not?

Sexuality is for most of our adult life very important to us. It makes us feel whole; reawakening of sexual behavior, when it has seemingly been lost, can continue to make us feel whole, and as a result, bring about further changes in sexual attitudes and behaviors.

Causes of Erectile Dysfunction

We have already discussed a number of the causes of male erectile dysfunction: diabetes, side effects of medications, physical limitations that limit mobility such as strokes or severe arthritis, congestive heart failure, and many more. But it has now become acceptable to discuss these matters and to seek to overcome the limitations. Certainly, the use of medication such as Viagra is one of these remedies. Other approaches include more vigorous treatment of underlying conditions such as diabetes, and more thorough rehabilitation after a heart attack or stroke. Please be aware, however, that the combined use of medications like nitroglycerin paste or tablets for the treatment of angina and the simultaneous use of Viagra are completely contraindicated; there is a dangerous drug-drug interaction between Viagra and nitroglycerine tablets that could prove fatal.

In terms of other medications causing undesirable sexual side effects, it is important to bring these to the attention of your doctor. You might be able to take a medication for blood pressure that does not have sexual side effects, or to replace antidepressant medications with psychotherapy if you are being treated for depression.

Factors Affecting Sexual Expression in Women

There are many factors affecting sexual activity in older women. As already mentioned, the most significant of these is the lack of available, sexually capable male partners. In other words, this includes women who are no longer married (widowed or divorced), and women who are still married but whose husbands are no longer sexually active. While there is a lot of discussion in the popular press about "cougars," that is, older women actively pursuing sexually active younger men, this concept generally relates to women in their 50s, not those in their 70s. The possibility of remarriage exists, as discussed in the chapter on social connections, but the numbers are stacked much more in the direction of an older man remarrying than of an older woman doing so.

Additional factors that tend to weigh against an older woman remaining sexually active are related to the fact that older women may now see themselves as less "sexy," or their partners see them as less attractive. Some women may experience pain during intercourse, due to thinned vaginal mucosa from lower estrogen levels, which can be remedied by the local application of estrogen creams. To date no such thing as "Viagra for women" has been developed.

How to Keep Your Sexual Life Alive

We now come to a discussion of what can be done to keep one's sexual life alive. There is little question in my mind, and in the minds of many others, that it is desirable to do so. Staying sexually active improves self-esteem. It improves closeness of the partners in a marriage or long-term relationship. It motivates both partners to do everything in their power to be attractive and appealing to their partner. This might also include the use of Botox to reduce forehead wrinkles or any variety of plastic surgery and well-toned muscles as a result of regular exercise. Maintaining good general health as well as mental health is also important. In fact it has been said that "good health is the ultimate aphrodisiac," and I am not one to disagree with that statement.

You can make adaptations that are designed to help you keep an active sexual life into your later years. Here are a few of these:

- Discuss any concerns you have about your sexual relationship with your partner, in an open, uncritical, and supportive way and be prepared to experiment to some degree with changes in the way you each express your sexuality.
- Discuss the same issues with your primary care doctor. By discussing your concerns openly with your doctor, you may be able to put him or her at ease, too.
- Yes, if you're physically able to (ask your doctor), do use Viagra or other medication to overcome erectile dysfunction, but remember that sexual stimulation is still needed, even with Viagra, for an erection to occur, and,

similarly, sexual stimulation is needed for the female partner to respond as well.

- Continue to take every opportunity to touch each other affectionately and supportively in your everyday contacts.
- Seek to replace any medications that interfere with sexuality with similar approaches that do not have this drawback. For example, antidepressant drugs can as easily interfere with the ability to enjoy sex.
- Emphasize intimacy over intercourse.
- Begin intimacy with touching, cuddling, kisses, holding hands, or massage, without regard as to whether it leads to intercourse or not.
- Consider satisfying each other through mutual masturbation when penetration does not seem possible.
- Be open to exploring oral sex, even if you have never considered this before. Even though the tongue is not a penis, it never suffers from erectile failure, and oral sex can be quite mutually satisfying.
- Use vaginal lubricants, such as K-Y Jelly or estrogen creams, if natural lubrication no longer occurs.
- Let your own imagination develop other variations that still provide you with intimacy and occasional sexual release.

Jeffrey and Edna were each widowed while living in the same retirement community. They each had had happy marriages that were sexually and emotionally fulfilling, and each missed their former partners very much. Neither of them thought they could ever replace their former partners. But as luck would have it, they both volunteered to work in a community agency that provides rides to persons needing to see their doctors, to go shopping, or to attend church services; he did so as a dispatcher, she as a volunteer driver. They found that they liked talking to each other over the phone. Then they met and had dinner together. Then they did it again. Then one of them expressed regret at having to go home to an empty house, even an empty bed. And lo and behold, they began to consider whether they could once again, after several years of abstinence, rekindle a sexual interest. And, bingo, it worked. They decided to live together, and after talking and thinking it over for some considerable time, they decided to remarry. They spoke to me of their new relationship in glowing terms. They came to truly love each other, including experiencing sexual intimacy. When on one occasion Jeffrey failed to experience an erection, Edna was very supportive and encouraged Jeffrey to talk to his doctor about Viagra. His doctor prescribed Cialis instead, but it worked miraculously well. And while they reported that they had sex only once or twice a week, it was clearly a high point in their relationship. In addition they found they liked each other very much, in other, various ways, and described their present marriage as "the dessert," while their previous marriages had been "the entrée."

Sexually Transmitted Diseases—a Cautionary Note

While I am encouraging older people to maintain an active sexual life and identity, I also need to ring a note of caution here. Advancing age does not reduce a person's vulnerability to sexually transmitted diseases, such as AIDS, syphilis, and gonorrhea. In fact, physicians and public health officials have become aware that STDs continue to be a significant risk for older people as well as for sexually active people of all ages. Thus, individuals entering upon new sexual relationships need to be equally cautious and prudent as at any age, to frankly discuss previous sexual relationships and other risk factors with prospective sex partners. Interesting, some advertisements for medications to treat erectile dysfunction now include warnings that these medications do not prevent sexually transmitted diseases.

Sex in the Nursing Home?

Yes, sex is even possible if your partner has been admitted to a nursing home, so long as your partner is willing and your nursing home is enlightened enough to provide you with privacy for a "conjugal visit." I mean, if convicted criminals are allowed conjugal visits, shouldn't you as a law-abiding citizen be allowed the same privilege? Of course, do this only if both partners are interested and willing.

So you see, sex is no different from anything else, only better. Live your life to the fullest, and that may involve being inventive and creative. As mentioned earlier, creativity counteracts aging.

Chapter Summary

- You are still a sexual being at any age.
- There is still a certain amount of taboo attached to sex among older people.
- Men and women continue to be interested in sexual expression.
- Understand erectile dysfunction in men.
- Since 1998 we have had Viagra.
- Know the factors that affect sexual expression in older women.
- Learn how to keep your sexual life alive.
- You may need to make modifications to keep your sexual life alive.
- Sex in the nursing home?
- Sex retards aging, if for no other reason than that is is also good exercise.

Chapter 14

Give Charitably, and Reap the Rewards

AT THIS STAGE of your life you probably have most of what you will ever need. The time for acquisitions is over; the time for distribution and dissemination is here. This is a special time given all that you possess: love, wisdom, advice, teachable skills, as well as tangible goods such as money, books, works of art, furniture, stocks and bonds, keepsakes of sentimental value, and more. The benefits to the giver are far greater than those of the receiver. This is your opportunity to leave a living legacy with family and friends, as well as religious, educational, artistic, community, or welfare organizations. Such acts of giving can in fact result in a kind of immortality, as the effect of charitable giving can live on for generations to come.

To quote Leeza Gibbons, television and radio person-ality: "The way we get to live forever is through memo-ries stored in the hearts and souls of those whose lives we touch. That is our soul print. It is our comfort, our nourishment at the end of the day and at the end of our life. How wonderful that memories can be called up at will and savored randomly. It seems to me we should spend our lives in a conscious state of creating these meaningful moments that live on. Memories matter."

I confess that changing from acquiring things to giv-ing away things may take some getting used to. Let me speak here from my personal experience. My wife and I have accumulated many books of all types: textbooks, novels, books of poetry, art books, cook books, travel books, dictionaries, books of advice, you name it. Most of our books are housed in our guesthouse, where they cover all of one long wall and a portion of another. Re-cently I have begun to invite every guest who has stayed with us to choose as many books as they might like and to take them with them as our gift. As you might guess, some of the first books to be taken away were some of my or my wife's favorites. It took real restraint and bit-ing our tongues to not go back on our invitation and ask our guest not to go away with this or that favorite book of ours. But it has gotten easier, and we truly feel joy now in seeing our books leave us to find new homes.

We have also begun to do the same with works of art and items of furniture as well. Again, there were initial hesitations, but it got easier and more joyful the more practiced we became in our giving. In addition, we regularly drop off bundles of unwanted or duplicate items at resale stores run by such charitable organizations as Goodwill, the Kidney Foundation, and a variety of others. Clothing, household goods, and furniture in good condition are much sought after and can be made available at little cost to persons in need. Part of the idea is to travel lighter, to unclutter, and to recycle.

Leave a Legacy

This issue requires a great deal of thought and research before you act, because it will determine the kind of legacy you leave behind for generations to come. I have always been impressed with the fact that Henry VIII endowed several scholarly chairs at Oxford University. With an endowment, the principal of the donation is never spent; but the interest generated by the principal provides benefits indefinitely. Thus Henry VIII's endowment is still providing funds for scholars at Oxford University to this date and will do so in perpetuity. Maybe you can be the next Henry VIII at your alma mater, minus the chopped-off heads. Here are two options available to you:

Gifts to Charitable Organizations Made during Your Lifetime

One instrument that is available to you is to make a gift annuity at your favorite charitable or educational organization. For contributing a certain sum, let us say $100,000, to your chosen organization, you will receive a lifetime income of approximately 5 to 6 percent of the gift amount, depending on your age at the time of your gift, or about $5,000 to $6,000 per year. Of this amount, a considerable portion will be paid to you tax-free, with the rest considered taxable income. In addition, you will receive a major charitable contribution deduction, or perhaps one-third of the gift amount, in the year that you make the donation. This will reduce your income tax liability substantially during the year of your gift. At the end of your life, or at the end of your spouse's life, the remaining principal in the annuity account will be applied to whatever charitable purpose you have designated: a scholarship, a building, or special innovative programs. In addition, you can have your name, or the name of someone you wish to honor, attached to the scholarship, building, or special program. This type of charitable contribution is also described in the chapter on preserving your wealth.

Another type of charitable gift you can make during your lifetime is a charitable remainder trust. This type of gift has similar benefits to you or your co-annuitant. You (and your co-annuitant) will receive an annuity for life. The residual will fund whatever program you have previously selected.

In as much as the gifts described here are complex, you should make these types of commitments only in consultation with a financial advisor who is thoroughly familiar with all aspects of charitable giving. Here is an example of what one couple did:

Calvin and Esther are a highly educated couple from a middle-class background who had grown up with limited resources except for the education their respective parents had provided them. They both worked in the field of medicine, he as a department head in the field of family medicine, and she as a nurse until their several children required her to spend more time at home. After they had gone off to college, she returned to some nursing work, but only as a volunteer. Along the way she became interested in investing, and her husband turned over a modest portion of his $100,000-plus salary for her to "play with" in the market.

Competitive as she had always been, she became remarkably successful in this endeavor, and over a period of some 20 years of investing had "grown" the several thousand dollars she received each year as "play money" into the remarkable sum of $4.5 million. So, as Calvin was approaching retirement, they decided together to donate a sizeable portion of their investments to the university for which they had both worked. They created an endowment to support scholarships for underprivileged students of nursing, a cause Esther had championed for years. About this time, at age 63, Esther was diagnosed with Alzheimer's disease.

Even though she was beginning to show signs of some impairment, they proceeded with their plans, as they had enough to live on as well as to provide care for Esther in the later stages of her disease. Esther was still able to participate in interviewing some of the scholarship candidates, which gave her enormous pleasure. The university honored them both by holding a special celebration when the first several students were awarded scholarships.

Some of the money Esther had cleverly invested continued to grow, even despite the "great recession of 2008." When Esther died in 2010, her husband further honored her by creating a research fund for Alzheimer's disease in her name. When he was asked why he continued to be interested in making charitable contributions, he said that he hoped that "the power of his example" might induce other individuals to also consider making end-of-life charitable contributions. The university continues to say thank you to Calvin in many ways. Calvin and Esther had also provided their children with an excellent professional education. As a result, the children supported their parents' generosity fully, as they were able to lead independent lives without needing to rely on any inheritance from their parents.

Gifts Made as Part of Your Will, or at the End of Your Life

For many, a will-based gift can often be much larger than one made during your lifetime. Such gifts can be in the form of money, appreciated stocks, bonds, real estate, or other valuables, such as art objects. Again, you can select how these gifts are to be spent, for which program or activity (scholarships, buildings, innovative programs that you select), or you can leave the use of the funds to the discretion of the organization to which you are contributing. Again, this may create naming opportunities, either in your or your partner's name, or in the name of someone you seek to honor. There's immortality for you! Here is another illustration:

> Ingrid was the caregiver for her mother, who suffered from pancreatic cancer. In her quest to get the best care for her mother for this nearly inoperable condition, she tried to seek out the most innovative, creative, and inventive surgeon. She located a surgeon who had just devised a new technique for dealing with this particular malignancy. As a result, her mother survived for five more years, when the usual remaining life expectancy for this condition would have been only about one year. In her gratitude, Ingrid wanted to honor her mother's surgeon by establishing an endowed chair to conduct further research in this complex surgical area. She offered to provide a gift of one-half of the amount required to establish an endowed chair, while the university and the

surgeon persuaded several other donors to complete this endowment. The university offered to name the chair in Ingrid's honor. Ingrid, however, modestly declined, insisting that the chair be named in honor of the surgeon who had treated her mother. This generous act of self-denial allowed other donors to come forward to complete the gift to establish an important research resource honoring the creative surgeon.

To the extent that these illustrations may have been meaningful to you I would say: "Go thou and do likewise."

Forgive Existing Debts

You may want to consider forgiving a debt owed to you by a relative, a former employee, or anyone else to whom you have extended credit. Children sometimes have been given loans to attend college or a professional school. It would indeed be an act of great generosity to simply forgive the debt owed to you. However, if a debt instrument exists between you and that debtor, you need to take the trouble to formally release the person from that debt. Again, consult with your financial advisor to do so in a manner that does not generate additional gift or estate taxes.

Forgive Those Who Have Offended You

Yet another charitable act you can engage in is to forgive any individual who has offended you, or against whom you may have been holding a grudge. You need not consult a financial advisor on this, but you might possibly consult your spiritual advisor on this type of gift giving. Your spiritual self will benefit greatly from any such act of forgiveness.

This might also be the best time to consider forgiving yourself for any acts of omission or commission that you regret, and to ask forgiveness of anyone whom you have offended. Again, your spiritual self will benefit greatly.

CHAPTER SUMMARY

- Make charitable giving your road to immortality.
- Be charitable now, and you will benefit.
- Unload and recycle in order to travel light.
- Forgive uncollected debts from relatives or friends.
- Forgive those who have offended you.
- Forgive yourself also for any acts of omission or commission.
- Ask and receive forgiveness from any one whom you may have offended.

Chapter 15

Plan for a Good Good-Bye

THINKING ABOUT one's own death is very personal. For many it has philosophical or religious meanings. Dying is natural. It happens to all living creatures. But during this last phase of our lives, thoughts about death have special importance. On the one hand, we are prepared for it; yet when it is imminent, it may cause another whole range of emotions.

Of course, we must accept the inevitability of death, and the fact that none of us will get out of this life alive. Accordingly, it comes down to *how* we are going to say good-bye. At least to a certain degree, our dying should be planned. We should decide ahead of time how we want our death to be handled, and let those close to us know our preferences. Do we want to be buried or cremated? Do we want there to be a funeral, memorial service, or a celebration of our life? We should have a plan for distributing our property. We should do so in an orderly, explicit fashion so as to minimize conflict, controversy, and possible pain. We should leave a legacy—it is up to each of us—how we want to be remembered. We should specify the kind of end-of-life care we would want for ourselves. We need to choose whether extraordinary means should be employed to keep us alive when there is no more hope for recovery, or whether we should just let nature take its course. To illustrate some of the issues involved, here is a brief vignette of what *not* to do:

> Ted was the owner of a successful hardware store. He was married and had two daughters. However, his marriage ran into difficulty and he divorced. After several years he remarried and had another daughter in that marriage. His business continued to be successful, and his two older daughters worked in his business, one providing accounting, and the other administrative services. Ted enjoyed the good life, liked to eat, drink, and smoke, and seemed to be comfortable and contented.
>
> Then he developed a persistent cough, and

on one occasion he coughed up blood. He went to see a doctor, had an X-ray of his chest, and learned that he had lung cancer. He sought treatment, but before long it became clear that the cancer had already spread to other parts of his body. He underwent radiation and chemotherapy, but the chemo made him feel ill and it was unable to contain the cancer, and he was thought to be incurable. When he was placed in hospice care, he complained that he didn't know why he was there. Since he never really accepted the fact that he was dying, he made no preparations for his death. He died without a will, leaving behind a wife and an ex-wife, two children from his first marriage and one from his second marriage, without any specifications as to how his business should be continued, or how his property should be divided. He also had a dog he loved very much, but he didn't make any provision for his care either. This resulted in acrimonious battles between his widow, his ex-wife, and his three children, leaving all of them intensely unhappy. A good deal of his wealth was dissipated in the cost of litigation. Clearly, denial is not the best way of preparing for death.

During the time leading up to your own death, you have the opportunity to attend many a funeral and many a memorial service. This may help you decide how you want to be remembered. In the meantime, concentrate on having a good life.

Create a Critical Information Folder

This "critical information folder" is for your family. It contains all of following:

- Location or copy of your most recent will.
- Location and key to your safe deposit box.
- Location or copy of your general and medical power of attorney
- Detailed description of all your real estate holdings, stocks and bonds, and other investment vehicles, as well as all bank or credit union accounts and any other assets you may hold.
- List all your liabilities and/or outstanding debts.
- Detailed description of all your retirement benefits as well as life insurance policies, including passwords to such accounts and beneficiary designations.
- Passwords to your computer accounts and to other important documents.
- A list of all your personal property items and how you would like to see them distributed to family members, friends, or charitable organizations.

- Your own suggested obituary. Don't make it too long, let it be a celebration of your life, and include a picture of yourself (smiling!).
- Specify who shall take care of your surviving pets.
- Indicate your preferences as to how you would like to be buried or cremated, and if, when, and how you would like to be memorialized.
- List your frequent flyer accounts and their passwords (did you know that your surviving spouse can request to have your frequent flyer miles transferred to his or her account by filling out an affidavit and enclosing a copy of your death certificate?).
- Anything else that you feel your survivors need to know.

One more thing: Don't make too big of a deal of your own death. Another poem may illustrate this point of view further:

Dying Is Nothing

dying is nothing
like I thought
no cymbals crashing
no illuminations
only deep
imperturbable
peace

None of us knows how we are going to die. We could die suddenly, in our sleep, in an accident, from a heart attack, a stroke, or a sudden cardiac irregularity. Or we could die at the end of a long illness. In the first case, we do not need to do anything specific at the time of our death, except to be ready for it to come at any time. But in the instance of dying after a long illness, how we manage our life during the course of the illness, right up to the final moment, does matter. We have choices to make: Avail ourselves of every treatment possible, including participating in experimental studies of treatments that have not yet been fully proven; or "let nature take its course" and allow currently available treatment to give us the best chance for extending our lives. Most important of all, however, is that you continue to engage with your doctors, that you fully understand what your treatment choices are, and that you continue to fully engage with your family, your friends, and your community, and that you not simply withdraw.

If and when the time comes that all possibilities for a cure have been exhausted, then you should take advantage of one of the most beneficial and humane approaches to oncoming death: hospice care.

Understand What Hospice Care Is

When you or someone in your family has reached the stage in medical care where full recovery is not possible and remaining life expectancy is judged to be no more than six months, hospice care can be instituted. Hospice care provides end-of-life care that is devoted to making the person comfortable. Those who are experiencing pain can be kept pain-free with a regimen of powerful medication, without concern about becoming addicted. Hospice care is perhaps most commonly used for patients with disseminated cancer. But it can also be used for someone in the late stages of Alzheimer's disease, heart disease, chronic obstructive pulmonary disease, or any other terminal condition. Care is provided either in the patient's own home or in a home-like setting. Psychological comfort and communication with family members and friends and religious or spiritual affiliations is emphasized. Importantly, hospice care is provided at no additional cost as a regular Medicare or Medicaid benefit.

Hospice services may include ongoing care by physicians, nurses, social workers, or mental health specialists. An important aspect of hospice care is that trained volunteers make up a significant part of the hospice personnel. Such volunteers can provide emotional support and companionship, carry out errands, or provide transportation.

A Final Note

At the end of a long and meaningful life, saying good-bye to those left behind should be done in the same manner as you have lived your life: with awareness, with dignity, with kindness and understanding, still loving and being loved, in your own signature way.

CHAPTER SUMMARY

- Learn to say good-bye with dignity.
- Create a "critical information folder" for your family that will facilitate their dealing with your departure.
- When cure is no longer possible, consider hospice care.
- Say good-bye as you have lived, in your own signature way.

Chapter 16

Know These Secrets of Successful Living

THANK YOU for having traveled with me this far. I would now like to share with you a few thoughts that are not related just to retirement. They are thoughts that have guided me throughout my life, and they may be of interest and value to you as well.

They don't by any stretch of the imagination amount to a coherent philosophy, but you could think of them as "philosophical," for want of a better word. My life has been graced by enormously good fortune. What success I've had I cannot take credit for. That credit belongs instead to a thousand people with whom I have come in contact, starting with my parents. My parents gave me good genes, for which I am truly grateful. They taught me the value of education, and they pinched pennies and denied themselves often in order to give me that good education. Much of what I know I learned from them: to be independent; to speak clearly; to be responsive; to listen; to take action. I owe them so much and I can never repay them except with love and praise in remembrance of them. I have dedicated this book to their memory.

There are others in my life who have taught me: teachers, bullies, gamblers, petty criminals (I never knew any big-time criminals), my girlfriends over the years before I met my wife of 46 years. To her I am extremely grateful. To her I can still show my gratitude while we are both alive. She has definitely had a hand in helping this book to come into being: She has read every word, every line, and every paragraph, over and over. She has made many suggestions that have improved the book in a major way, to the point where she might be considered a virtual co-author, although she has declined that honor. So here is to her: An enormous "Thank you!"

In the next section you will find selected quotes, followed by my personal comments concerning each of them. These quotes come from many differing sources: philosophers, philosophies, authors, poets, scientists, ordinary citizens, and general life lessons. I have chosen not to attribute each of them, and they are certainly not mine. They are quotes that I have found to be valuable and valid in guiding my life. I hope they may also prove valuable to you. For those of you who insist on knowing the source of these quotes, I recommend that you Google them. You will find one or even many differing origins for the majority of them.

"Everything is connected to everything else."

Everything and everyone is connected to everything and everyone else. Every change here brings about changes there. Our past actions have influenced our current ones; one chain of events is connected to all other events. We are all made of the same stuff; we are all humans. There are no strangers, and there are no enemies. One act of kindness leads to other acts of kindness, and the opposite is also true. We are all part of the whole. We are all responsible.

"Every day is a gift."

Every day is a new beginning. At the beginning it is perfect. All possibilities are open. So try not to mess it up. Give thanks for where the day takes you. Give love every moment. With that you can't go wrong.

"The only moment you have is now."

The present is your present. This is the only moment you have, and what you do in this moment matters most. So be attentive and aware of what you are thinking, feeling, and doing in this one moment. The past is past. The future cannot be foreseen. But in this moment, you need to do the right thing, do it now, and do it with the people you are with, for this is what you will be held accountable for. *Carpe diem!*

"To get what you want, help other people get what they want."

I don't have much to say about this saying except "try it!"

"Connect with the creative and the curative nature of nature."

If ever you despair of trying to find perfection among human beings, give nature a try. There you will see perfection in endless ways, in orchids, in oak trees, in the sky, in the breeze you feel, in the oceans, in wild animals. Not only can the experience of everyday nature fill you with awe, but it can also be tremendously soothing and healing to whatever pain you might be experiencing.

"God writes all the books."

The above statement does not require that you believe in God. It is used here to indicate how creativity proceeds more or less on its own. Those of us who want to be creative, whether it be in words, or music, or color, or form, such as in sculpture or architecture, are drawn to do so by a vision of what we want to create: a poem, a symphony, a painting, a building, or a clay sculpture. If we know what we want to achieve, we need only to proceed in the direction we want to go, and allow the actions to flow as they may (we can make corrections later), but the act of creativity is to some degree automatic, driven by forces we may fail to understand, but proceeding nevertheless to attain our vision. All we have to do is listen and put pen to words. The words will all come. We don't have to do a thing.

"Let kindness be your religion."

The Dalai Lama, during one of his trips to the United States, said that kindness was his religion. He emphasized the important role that compassion plays in bringing about inner peace. He also teaches that compassion has to be learned, practiced over and over again, until it becomes a habit. We could do worse than to follow his advice.

"Endings are also beginnings."

Nothing ever ends; it just leads to other things, other experiences. For every door that closes, another one opens. For every chapter that ends, a new chapter begins. While endings are sometimes sad, they also bring new opportunities, new relationships, and new ideas. When you come to an ending, turn the page, close the book, and go on to the next one. It might be even more interesting or more rewarding than the one you have finished.

The poem below was written on my last day at work, just before heading off to my staff retirement party, where I read the poem out loud, and almost cried.

Endings Are Beginnings

Today I saw my final patient.
Fifty years ago I saw my first.
What did I feel? Triumph?
Sorrow? Emptiness?
Only this: One door closes,
one door opens.
Endings are beginnings.
I begin again:
a whole generation left to live,
failure ruled out by definition,
all possibilities are open,
nothing more to prove.
I get in my car and drive home.
Rain is starting to fall.
Today I saw my final patient.
My dog welcomes me just the same.

"Be imperturbable."

Imperturbable peace lies deep within you. You can access your own stillness almost anywhere, at any time, even in the midst of turmoil and stress. Take a few deep breaths, quiet your mind, and let that delicious stillness fill you. Blame nothing on anyone else. Life has its seasons, and it has its seesaws. There is no chain of disasters that will not come to an end. This, too, shall pass. Be imperturbable.

"Forgive, and keep on forgiving; that includes forgiving yourself."

To forgive those who have offended us, hurt us, or slighted us is a precious commodity of which we have a potentially endless supply. Not only does forgiving our friends, relatives, or even enemies end painful feelings within ourselves, it lays the groundwork for positive relationships in the future. Nowhere is this more true than in forgiving yourself. If you have felt unhappy with yourself for having done something or for failing to have done what you should have done, forgiving yourself clears the path to doing better from here on out.

"The job of every cell in the body is to nourish and support every other cell."

And that is our job, too: to nourish all those with whom we come in contact. We are all in this together. Any good we do will benefit everyone. Any evil we do will harm everyone. As we sow, so shall we reap.

"Beware the law of unintended consequences."

The law of unintended consequences states that even acts that are well-meant and well thought-out can have unintended consequences. This advice, then, is to look out for the possibility of such events. An example of this might be the effect of treatment with anti-inflammatory steroids for diseases of inflammation, such as rheumatoid arthritis, leading to osteoporosis or the onset of diabetes. Another example is the benefit of the invention of the automobile leading to air pollution.

"Creativity retards aging."

Creating something new not only creates a new product, or art, or writing, but it also enhances our self-esteem. It is remarkable how long-lived creative people are, and the creation of works of art can be one of the things you may wish to experience in retirement.

"Whenever you visit anyone, bring them a gift."

The pleasure that comes from giving is far greater than that which comes from receiving. Whenever you visit anyone, bring a gift. It could be something mate-rial, such as a book, a picture, a bouquet of flowers, a favorite dish you have prepared, or a bottle of wine. But it could also be something less tangible such as congratulations, good wishes, a compliment, an ex-pression of affection, or gratitude for your friendship with that person. You will be amply rewarded for your generosity by the good feelings it will give you. Often you may even receive a gift, or a compliment, in return. But you will find your real reward in the giving, not the receiving.

"Such is the rapture of wine that the sober shall never inherit."

This is a quote from the Chinese poet Li Po, who ex-tols the virtues of drinking wine in the company of friends. This should not be viewed as an encourage-ment of drunkenness, but drinking with friends in moderation can definitely be rewarding. In fact, I was so impressed with the poems of this ancient poet, that early on in my life I wrote a poem in his honor, the title of which became the title of my first published book, a book of poems. I share the poem with you here:

Take with Me Now That Enormous Step, Li Po
In the clean morning air
I put aside at last
pages and pages of Li Po.
We have been drinking partners,
comrades for a night
in the drunkenness of words,
in a bed across ages,
alive to the same air
from here to China.
Take with me now
that enormous step,
Li Po, into sleep.

The Most Powerful Words in the World:

"I need your help."

There are no phrases more magical than this one. This is one of the most powerful phrases in the human language, bested perhaps only by "I love you." Just like with the phrase "I love you," don't be afraid to use it. No one ever minds being asked for help. No one ever minds being told that they are loved. Use it only when you really need the help of someone else, which will happen often enough in your lifetime. Rarely will you be turned down. After all, how would you respond if someone asked for your help? Also, ask intelligently, precisely, and specifically for what you need. That will make it easier to for you to get the exact help you need.

"I love you."

Never be afraid to use it when it is true. Never use it when it is not. Say it to men, women, and children. You can even say it to pets, and they will understand.

"I am truly sorry."

Learn to use this phrase whenever it applies.

"Thank you."

No one will ever mind being thanked. More often it is the failure to say "thank you" that will be noticed.

"You are amazing!"

This is a little phrase that I have learned to use, because the few times someone said that to me, it really made me proud, and I've always remembered it, with a huge amount of gratitude for the person who said it.

"Congratulations!"

Congratulations are always in order when someone you care about has accomplished something. Tell them you're proud of them, tell them you are pleased for them, and show them that you have taken notice. All you need to do is to remember how good it felt when someone said "congratulations" to you. Don't let the opportunity go by unused.

CHAPTER SUMMARY

- Everything is connected to everything else.
- Every day is a gift: Live life every day.
- To get what you want help other people get what they want.
- Connect with the creative and the curative nature of nature every day.
- Realize that God writes all the books.
- Endings are also beginnings.
- Be imperturbable.
- Forgive, and keep on forgiving. And that includes forgiving yourself.
- Be aware of the law of unintended consequences.
- Creativity retards aging.
- Whenever you visit anyone, bring a gift.
- Such is the rapture of wine that the sober shall never inherit.
- Know and use the most powerful words in the world.

A to Z Nuggets of Information

In this appendix you'll find brief discussions of interesting topics that affect the elderly. The topics are arranged alphabetically. You may just want to skim these pages or read the entire section, since any of these items could become relevant to you or family members and friends at one time or another during your retirement years.

Addiction to Pain Medications

Elderly patients are prone to experience pain from arthritis, as a result of earlier life accidents or injuries, diabetic neuropathy, or post-herpetic neuropathy (post-shingles neuropathy, also see Zoster infections in this section). Naturally such individuals will seek relief. They may try various over-the-counter pain relievers such as aspirin, Tylenol, or other non-steroidal medications, but they may find that these do not bring complete relief. They may therefore be drawn to doctors who are pain specialists or to specialized pain clinics. These individuals may be given more powerful pain relievers, generally medications that are derivatives or analogues of codeine or morphine. Drugs in this category are numerous indeed and may include Darvocet, Percocet, hydrocodone, OxyContin, and many others. These latter drugs are not only highly effective but they are also highly addictive. The person using them may develop tolerance to them, requiring higher and higher doses to get the same amount of pain relief. The prescribing doctor may resist increasing either the dosage or frequency of the drug, fearing addiction. Unfortunately, pain specialists and pain clinics are now much advertised, and individuals with chronic pain may be tempted to go to more than one doctor or clinic to get additional medication. And thus the addiction process begins.

Addiction to pain medication in the elderly is as serious a problem as addiction to so-called recreational drugs in younger persons. Unless a strong-minded primary care doctor is involved and aware of all the medications the patient is taking, the addiction process is likely to continue. As with other addictions, an "intervention" may need to be staged to begin the process of correction. This can be effective when the patient, the family, and all the doctors involved cooperate, so that the patient receives consistent feedback about the need for drug withdrawal, and subsequent tight control of pain medication under the care of only a single prescribing doctor. Of course, finding a remedy for the cause of the continuing pain would be the best solution.

AIDS (HIV) and Sexually Transmitted Diseases

It used to be that HIV (human immunodeficiency virus) was primarily a concern for younger people, but that is no longer true. The risk for acquiring HIV is not at all diminished as one gets older. So, to the extent that you are at sexually active, it is necessary that you know the HIV status of your sexual partner. Nor is it the only sexually transmitted disease (STD) that you need to be concerned about, especially as it relates to any new sexual partner. The use of condoms with any new sexual partner is strongly recommended. For those of you who are simply continuing an ongoing monogamous sexual relationship, you should have smooth sailing.

Arthritis

Arthritis, especially osteoarthritis, is probably the most common disease affecting older people. Osteoarthritis can affect any of the joints in your body, fingers, toes, hips, and knees, even the spine. Pain is the predominant symptom, with limitation of motion a close second. Your primary care doctor is probably the best person to advise you on what combination of pain medication and exercise (the two key treatment elements for osteoarthritis) you need to apply. Treatment rather depends on the location and severity of your arthritis. Unfortunately, medical science has not yet discovered any cure for this common condition. It is important that you achieve a relatively pain-free status, with little or no limitation of motion.

Audio Books

Audio books are a wonderful way to enjoy books of every kind: fiction, non-fiction, biography, what have you. You can listen to audio books while driving, while on an airplane or on a cruise, and while doing ordinary household chores. Listening makes the time fly and relieves boredom. Audio books can be enjoyed even with visual difficulties, and they are easier to carry around than books. Your local library and bookstore have them available in a plentiful supply. So, enjoy!

Bathroom Safety

Your bathroom is where you are most likely to experience an accident or fall. So fall-proof this room in your house by installing handrails at your bathtub, and by avoiding throw rugs that can slide easily under your feet. Most important, make sure your bathroom floors are always dry before you step on them. Wet bathroom floors are slicker than ice. And even if you now live in an area where ice is no longer a problem, wet bathroom floors can do as much damage as ice.

Berries

Of all the delicious foods you may consume, berries of every kind are probably the most nutritious for you. They contain significant amounts of antioxidants.

This goes for blueberries, strawberries, raspberries, and every other kind of berry you can think of. I recently planted a whole string of blueberries to have my own supply at hand, more or less year-round. But even if you don't grow them in your own yard, remember it is "always summer somewhere," and that means that berries are available from somewhere even when none are ripening here in the United States. Chile and other South American countries are a great source of berries in winter, and although a little pricey at those times, they are well worth it in terms of taste and health benefits.

Blood in the Urine, Coughing Up Blood, Black or Tarry Stools, or Rectal Bleeding

The presence of blood in any bodily excretion such as urine, stools, or sputum usually indicates a serious medical condition and requires prompt medical attention. Blood in the urine may be caused by kidney or bladder stones, or by a tumor in the bladder or the kidney. Coughing up blood can be an indicator of a possible tumor of the lungs or the bronchial system, and tarry stool may indicate bleeding from any part of the gastrointestinal system. Thorough medical tests are needed to pinpoint the cause of the bleeding and to correct the disease causing the bleeding.

Botox

Increasingly, both women and men are taking advantage of the benefits of Botox injections and facial plastic surgery to improve their appearance. Botox injections reduce facial lines, while facial plastic surgery, or "face lifts," can make people appear as young as they feel. The stigma that was once attached to such procedures has all but disappeared, and costs as well as the time required for these procedures have been markedly reduced. As a result, they are now available to more and more people.

Books for the Blind

Books for the Blind is a federally funded program available to persons with partial as well as complete impairment of vision. Books can be delivered to eligible readers postage-free and can be returned in the same manner. Thus people who cannot read any longer due to visual impairment can still enjoy the content of books by hearing them read by professional readers, and sometimes by the authors themselves. Special cassette players for this program can also be borrowed without charge. Contact your local library for information to get you started.

Bowel Problems: Constipation, Diarrhea

Bowel problems, especially constipation, are notorious for plaguing the lives of older people. But here, again, there *is* something you can do about them. Exercising and eating fresh fruits and vegetables are quite effective in preventing constipation. If diarrhea ever troubles you for more than a few episodes, it is important that you maintain adequate fluid intake to replace lost fluids. Effective anti-diarrhea medications are available in your local drug stores. Any continued occurrence of diarrhea requires medical evaluation as to the cause.

Breast Cancer

Breast cancer requires special attention. The reasons for this are numerous and complex. First, it is one of the most common forms of cancer in women. Second, early diagnosis and treatment are more significant in this form of cancer than in almost any other cancer because (1) frequent self-exams are one of the best means available for early discovery; and (2) regularly performed mammography (X-ray examination of the breasts) can also detect this cancer in its early stages. Third, cancer of the breast, including treatment of breast cancer, has perhaps the greatest impact on the affected person's self-image and self-esteem. Fourth, multiple treatment options need to be considered when breast cancer is discovered, ranging from lumpectomy (simple surgical excision of the tumor) to simple mastectomy, radical mastectomy, bilateral mastectomy, radiation, and/or chemotherapy. The differential benefit and impact of each of these procedures requires truly expert as well as complex personal decision-making. Accordingly, when breast cancer is discovered, treatment should optimally take place in one of the nationally recognized and federally funded cancer centers.

Affected individuals should not only consider standard treatments but also explore the availability of newer, experimental forms of treatments as well. DNA testing is also available for a particularly dangerous form of inherited breast cancer tendency. This is especially significant if there is a strong family history of breast cancer.

Cancer

Cancer may well be one of the most feared words in the English language, second only perhaps to Alzheimer's. The basic approach to dealing with the possibility of cancer is to maintain regular medical checkups with your primary care physician and an awareness of the early warning signs of cancer: any abnormal growth, bleeding from any bodily orifice, bone pain, or abnormal weight loss for which no other cause has been found. Cancer can best be treated if it is discovered early. It can be excised surgically from most sites of the body. Where it cannot be removed surgically, chemotherapy and radiation therapy are now available. One additional hint: If you are dealing with cancer, put yourself under the care of an oncology specialist and be open to the possibility of participating in clinical trials of new medications if no established treatments exist.

Also understand that basal cell and squamous cell cancers of the skin are generally not invasive, although they still require removal. Cancer of the prostate is a very different kind of cancer, in that it almost always grows very slowly. Consult with experts in prostate cancer to explore non-invasive treatments, or no treatments at all. For prostate cancer, an effective blood test is available, the PSA test, which will alert you and your doctor to your risk for prostate cancer.

Caregiving

It may well be that some of you will become caregivers to someone you love. A caregiver is person who cares for an individual who has become sick or disabled, usually with a chronic illness. That person may be a spouse, a close friend, or sometimes a parent or even an adult child. Caregiving is an intense, demanding, challenging activity, one for which most of you will be unprepared. Yet it can be a rewarding and satisfying activity as well. A caregiver needs to learn a great deal about the nature of the illness or the specific disability that occasions the caregiving. But he or she may need to learn a great deal about the nature of caregiving as well.

Chronic Pain

There are two great disadvantages that come from chronic pain: (1) pain hurts, obviously, and may limit your enjoyment of life, as well as your mobility; and

(2) chronic treatment with pain medication can lead to addiction. Accordingly, you need to do everything that you and your doctor can think of to remedy the cause of your chronic pain, and secondly, if you should require ongoing pain medications, do so only under the care of your primary care doctor rather than consulting multiple doctors. Since individuals suffering from chronic pain are at risk for addiction to pain medication, consult the section on addiction to pain medications earlier in this appendix and in the text. The only situation in which you need not be concerned about addiction to pain medication is if you are receiving pain medication for pain due to terminal cancer under the care of a hospice or palliative care physician.

Cruises

Ocean cruises are highly recommended for people in their retirement. They constitute an all-inclusive vacation in a wonderfully social environment. They come in all shapes and sizes, and often cater to special-interest groups. They may include lectures and other intellectual entertainment, travel to exotic places, and stopovers at many on-land sites. They can also be quite economically priced, if you search the Internet for advantageous rates or last-minute availabilities.

Diabetic Neuropathy

Diabetic neuropathy is a very serious complication of diabetes. It is the destruction of sensory nerves in the extremities, primarily the legs, caused by excessively high levels of glucose. Symptoms include a tingling sensation in the legs, leg pains, and decreased ability to sense stimuli in the affected areas. Tight control of glucose levels can prevent and minimize neuropathy, or even restore intact nerve function. Individuals with diabetic neuropathy are at risk for complications from even small injuries, as pain goes unnoticed and may lead to serious infections, even gangrene, which can require amputation of the affected part of the limb.

Drug-Drug Interactions

Drug-drug interactions become a concern when you are taking multiple medications for multiple health problems. Again, your primary care doctor, who is or should be aware of *all* of the medications you are taking, is in the best position to advise you of any possible drug-drug interaction. Remember that over-the-counter medications are just as likely as prescription medications to cause drug-drug interactions, so you need to be sure that your doctor knows about those, too.

Drug-drug interactions may be of two kinds: those in which two drugs taken together can enhance the risk of producing a side effect; and those drugs which, when taken together, will counteract the effect of one another. Any unexplained symptoms that you encounter following the addition of one more medication to what you are already taking should alert you and your doctor to the possibility of a drug-drug interaction. Alternative drugs can be prescribed for the condition being treated that do not have the particular drug-drug interaction in question.

Ear Problems

The most common ear problems in older people are the loss of hearing and decreased hearing acuity caused by damage to the auditory nerve. A thorough hearing evaluation is in order when someone begins to have hearing difficulty. There are very sophisticated hearing aids currently available that correct only those aspects of your hearing that have been damaged. Loss of hearing severely impairs communication and should be corrected if at all possible. Failure to correct hearing loss leads to social isolation, misunderstanding, and sometimes to paranoid reaction when a person misinterprets something that they did not hear completely or correctly. Hearing loss may become more common as the current generation of baby boomers, who were frequently exposed to very loud music, comes of age.

Eye Diseases: Cataracts, Glaucoma, Macular Degeneration, and Diabetic Retinopathy

The loss of vision is one of the most troubling aspects of getting older. The most common causes of vision loss are cataracts, glaucoma, macular degeneration, and diabetic retinopathy. Fortunately, treatments are now available for cataracts and glaucoma, and there are preventive measures for the other two. Cataracts are a thickening of the ocular lens with advancing age, leading to blurry or no vision. Cataracts can be removed surgically, and new lenses can be implanted. Glaucoma is an abnormally high pressure of the fluid inside the eyeball, which can be caused by age, and occasionally as a side effect of some medications. Medications, which must be used daily, are available to reduce the intraocular pressure, and older individuals should have eye examinations to check for these disorders either once a year or when symptoms occur. Macular degeneration is caused by the degeneration of the optic nerve cells inside the eye, and treatments for this condition are currently being developed. Diabetic retinopathy is a complication of poorly controlled diabetes. It is manifested by dilation of blood vessels inside the eye, which can be treated by laser ophthalmologic surgery. However, the best approach is to insist on tight control of diabetes and an annual eye examination that includes dilation of the iris by an ophthalmologist for a clear view of the back of the eye.

Fibromyalgia

Fibromyalgia is a condition that can occur at any age, but it can also appear for the first time in one's later years. It is characterized by widespread pain in muscles and joints, tenderness over multiple points of the body, and extreme fatigue. The cause of the condition is not entirely understood. It can best be treated through stress reduction, gentle exercise of the affected areas, and to some degree, by pain medication. Because it does not readily yield to treatment with pain medications, it can lead to possible addiction to pain medication, which then becomes an additional problem. Fibromyalgia is more common in women than in men. A number of non-pain medications, such as antidepressant medications, have been shown to be somewhat beneficial to those who have this disease.

Fish Oil

Fish oil, containing omega-3 fatty acids as well as DHA (docosahexaenoic acid) antioxidants, is probably the most universally agreed-upon supplement to be taken by people as they grow older. It has definite benefits in lowering the risk of coronary heart disease and of lowering blood cholesterol levels. Most people should take 1,000 mg daily, while those at greater risk of coronary heart disease, such as those with diabetes or high blood pressure, should take 2,000 mg per day. While you may see quite a bit of advice about taking just the "right" kind of fish oil, advice which no doubt has some merit, it is far more important that you take any fish oil that contains at least 200 mg of omega-3 and 200 mg of DHA. There are relatively few side effects from taking fish oil, but it can cause easy bruising of the skin in some people. If this occurs, the dose should be reduced to no more than 500 mg daily, and if the effect persists, it should probably be discontinued altogether. I personally take two 1,000-mg fish oil capsules daily and have been doing so for a number of years.

Geriatric Care Managers

A geriatric care manager is a relatively new type of professional who manages the care of an elderly person when that person does not have a relative or a close friend who can take on this role. He or she functions in general *in the place of a family caregiver,* when no family member is available or able to provide such care. Care managers are paid to organize, supervise, and coordinate social, health, and mental health services on behalf of aging persons. This may involve taking the patient to the doctor, getting medications from a drug store, and taking the patient to rehabilitation appointments. Geriatric care managers are generally either social workers or nurses, and they need to have a multidisciplinary orientation. No specific credentialing methods or standards exist as of yet for taking on the role and title of a geriatric care manager. The person responsible for employing a geriatric care manager has to rely on references, personal interviews, and reputation in selecting a care manager. This may have to be done at long-distance, as this kind of situation arises most often when the responsible family member lives in one location and the person requiring care lives in another location. Occasional personal contacts with the geriatric care manager are strongly recommended so that the decision-maker about care can be assured that appropriate care is indeed being delivered.

Home Health Care

A number of chronic health conditions may require the use of home health care following either hospitalization or surgery, or when such care is better delivered in the person's own home rather than in a hospital or doctor's office. It is usually nurses, physical therapists, or occupational therapists who deliver home health care, under the direction of the prescribing doctor. Frequently, home health care is covered under the patient's health care policy.

E-readers and E-books
(Kindle, Sony Reader, and Nook)

E-readers offer a new generation of electronic devices or programs for those who no longer can or wish to read printed books or magazines. These include Kindle, produced by Amazon.com; the Sony Reader, Nook, produced by Barnes and Noble; and other similar devices, including the Apple iPad. E-readers are particularly useful to people who cannot easily get to the library or bookstore. E-readers also have the advantage of being able to hold hundreds of books, which can thus be taken anywhere, on airplanes or cruises. Many people especially appreciate the fact that they can easily enlarge or shrink the print size, and new books can be downloaded electronically quickly and easily. You won't need much instruction to be able to use any of these devices with ease.

Loss of Sense of Taste and Smell

Losing the sense of taste and smell occurs to some degree in people of advanced age. This is regrettable, since it can diminish the enjoyment of foods and limit the food you might choose to eat. The sense of taste for sweets almost never disappears. Unfortunately, I can't give you any great remedy for this problem, so I can only commiserate with you if you are so affected. Sometimes malnutrition can result from the loss of enjoyment of a variety of foods; if you suspect this is a problem for you, you should consult with a dietician to make sure you're maintaining adequate caloric intake and balanced nutrition.

Malnutrition

As explained above, a certain degree of malnutrition can occur as a result of losing your sense of taste and smell late in life. More commonly, however, malnutrition is associated with a serious illness, such as cancer, a gastrointestinal disorder, or Alzheimer's disease. You should consult with a dietician to learn how to change your eating habits to assure adequate caloric intake and to avoid lowering overall resistance to disease.

Meditation

Meditation is the practice of focusing your attention to help you feel calm and give you intense awareness about your life. While largely developed in the Far East, it has now become a significant tool for wellness in western society as well. The practice focuses on your breathing and on awareness of what is happening in your mind right now, to the exclusion of worries or concerns about the past or the future. You can be taught meditation, or you can learn it from written descriptions of meditation technologies. Meditation has been shown to ameliorate anxiety states and pain. It can also be used to manage day-to-day stress and to produce deep relaxation without the use of medications.

Meditation involves sitting quietly for at least 15 to 20 minutes while concentrating on deep, relaxed breathing. Meditation is usually used in addition to conventional methods of treatment for the specific disease or condition. It is free of any side effects, and multiple studies have shown that it is beneficial in treating hypertension, anxiety, depression and pain syndromes, among others.

Nuts

After berries, which are covered earlier in this appendix, nuts are second in playing a very important role in a balanced, heart-healthy diet. Ideally, they should become a regular part of your diet. Nuts contain monounsaturated fatty acids (MUFAs), which tend to lower LDL cholesterol, the so-called bad cholesterol. They themselves contain no cholesterol. They are a good source of vegetable protein and fiber. They contain antioxidants as well as a number of important vitamins and minerals. Almonds, cashews, hazelnuts, macadamia nuts, peanuts, pecans, and walnuts are all delicious, and you can choose among all of these for variety. Although nuts are high in calories due to their fat content, they have a high satiety value, meaning that they quickly provide us a sense of fullness. Because of their calorie count, they should be eaten in relatively small quantities. However, they are versatile in that they can be eaten as snacks or as part of a meal, such as additions to cereals, salads, baked breads, and muffins, as well as to a variety of meat dishes. Vegetarians can enjoy them because they constitute a nearly complete food nutritionally. But you don't have to be a vegetarian to enjoy their taste and their health benefits.

Organ Transplants

Heart, liver, lung, and kidney transplants have become a possible means for replacing complex organs that are no longer functioning properly. But this is a much more complex process than a hip or a knee replacement. Organ transplants require a careful serological match between the donor and the future recipient. Organ donation must be planned in advance and takes advantage of the sad fact that some individuals will die in automobile accidents, for example, with perfectly intact organs. Even those dying from major disease may have organs that can still serve another individual for a good number of years. And since we are provided with two kidneys, it is possible for someone to donate one kidney to another individual, while still alive. In individuals who donate one kidney, their remaining kidney will grow to take over virtually all of the functions of the missing kidney. Another "live" organ transplant that is possible is a bone marrow transplant that can extend the life span of someone afflicted with leukemia. Again, the remaining bone marrow in the donor is quite sufficient to produce all the blood elements he or she will need while offering hope and extending life for another human being.

So, you may wish to consider signing up for organ donation at the time of your eventual death, whether it be an accidental or a natural one. On the other hand, if disease destroys *your* liver, kidneys, heart, or lungs, you may be eligible to be the beneficiary of organ donation and organ transplantation.

Osteoporosis

Osteoporosis is a serious bone disease. It is the loss of bone mass from vital bone structures, such as the spine, the hip, the knee, or the bones in the arms or legs. It is more common in older women than in older men, but it occurs in both. Osteoporosis has some degree of hereditary predisposition, but it can also come about from inadequate dietary intake of calcium and Vitamin D, from disuse, or from medications such as corticosteroids, which reduce bone formation and bone replacement. The bones of those who have osteoporosis are easily fractured from falls or trauma, and sometimes fractures occur spontaneously when the bones of the vertebral column have become so weak that they cannot support the weight of the body even at rest. Spinal fractures are both painful and disabling and require both immediate treatment of the fracture, such as by vertebroplasty or kyphoplasty, and treatments designed to restore increased bone formation. A number of such medications are currently available for the treatment of osteoporosis, in either weekly or monthly doses. Best known among osteoporosis medications are Fosamax, Actonel, and Boniva.

Parkinson's Disease

Parkinson's disease is a neurodegenerative disease affecting people with advancing age. It is characterized by stiff muscles, slowed muscle response, and a gross tremor that may affect the hands, the legs, and portions of the face. The tremor is most pronounced when the muscles are at rest, and it disappears or diminishes when the muscles are moved voluntarily. The stiffness of the facial muscles gives the affected individual a mask-like appearance. The voice is also affected, becoming low in volume and devoid of normal modulation.

If you experience these symptoms, you should be evaluated by your primary care doctor. While your primary care doctor can manage many aspects of Parkinson's disease, you should consult at least once with a neurologist in order to confirm the diagnosis and discuss treatment options.

As with a number of other neurodegenerative disorders, such as Alzheimer's disease, the exact cause of Parkinson's disease is not known. However, its symptoms are based on the loss of brain cells in the part of the brain that controls muscle movements. There may be a certain amount of hereditary risk for Parkinson's disease, so that *your* chances of developing the disease are slightly increased if a blood relative, such as your parent or sibling, has or had the disease. But as is true with other neurodegenerative diseases, age is the greatest risk factor.

While there is currently no cure for Parkinson's disease, a great deal is known about the disease that can help to slow its progression. We know that the loss of dopamine-producing cells leads to a deficit of this chemical, which is necessary for normal muscle function. The various treatments currently available are aimed at increasing the levels of dopamine in the brain, thereby reducing the severity of symptoms. Levodopa is the most effective treatment for the symptoms of Parkinson's disease, and it can initially result in remarkable improvement of symptoms. Over time, however, its effectiveness decreases. Then levodopa is usually combined with a drug called carbidopa, which slows the breakdown of levodopa. The combined drug is called Sinemet. As the disease progresses, higher and more frequent doses of Sinemet may need to be used. But over time, these higher doses may themselves lead to significant side effects. A more recent addition to the treatment program is a series of drugs called dopamine agonist, that is drugs that mimic the effect of the naturally occurring dopamine, including the brands Requip and Mirapex. These drugs may have a much longer period of effectiveness, but they are not nearly as efficient in controlling the tremors in Parkinson's disease. Research is under way in laboratories worldwide to find still more effective treatments for this disease.

In the late stages of Parkinson's disease, the affected individual will also develop memory loss and other symptoms of dementia, resembling those seen in Alzheimer's disease. Interestingly enough—though it is small comfort to the affected patients—is the fact that late in Alzheimer's disease, many patients will additionally develop symptoms of Parkinson's.

Plastic Surgery

"Having some work done," that is, plastic surgery, especially facial plastic surgery, is becoming more commonplace for both women and men, and especially in women and men who occupy highly visible or public positions. It can be a wonderful birthday present that you can give yourself or to your spouse. The risks of such surgery are minimal, and the improved appearance of signs of aging, such as loose skin folds about the face and neck, can make you both look and feel younger.

Podiatry

Both the feet and the hands are very complex structures, and care of the feet, especially in older people, may require a foot specialist, or a podiatrist. Individuals with diabetes are probably those with greatest risk for developing foot problems (see diabetic neuropathy in this appendix). In the diabetic patient with neuropathy it may be best to ask a podiatrist to trim toenails, as any small knick or cut to the foot can have drastic consequences. Infection can easily arise, easily spread, and can only be treated with difficulty. On a personal level, the diabetic patient needs to assure that his feet are always clean and dry, especially between the toes, as serious infections can begin in these close spaces when they remain wet. Podiatry is a subspecialty of surgery, and it is a podiatrist who would treat problems of the foot, ankle, and lower leg. This could include foot infections as well as areas of ulceration at the ankle and the lower legs, particularly occurring in diabetic patients. The lower part of the leg is only poorly supplied with the blood vessels that would promote healing, and diabetes further compromises the blood supply to the feet. Expert treatment of any foot infection or ankle ulceration is aimed at avoiding even more serious complications such as gangrene, which could lead to the need for amputation. Podiatrists can also provide the appropriate care for corns and calluses on the feet. Again, especially in diabetic patients, such care should be left to a podiatrist. Self care of such lesions in diabetic patients may lead to aggravated infections and is therefore to be avoided.

Prostate Problems

With advancing age, men may face one of two types of prostate problems: benign prostatic hypertrophy and cancer of the prostate. Both are troublesome and both require serious medical attention.

Benign prostatic hypertrophy is characterized by excessive growth of the prostate, an organ that surrounds the neck of the urinary bladder. The vast majority of older men will experience this excessive growth. As the prostate enlarges, it can impair the flow of urine from the bladder, leading to a slowed urinary stream, increased daytime and nighttime urinary frequency, and incomplete bladder emptying. If these symptoms are not heeded and the problem not attended to, a more dramatic event will occur: complete bladder shut down, resulting in severe pain in the bladder area from an overfilled bladder. Emergency catheterization is performed to overcome the problem. Fortunately there are now several medications available to alleviate these problems. One is a drug that inhibits the growth of the prostate and reduces an already enlarged prostate. The other is a drug that permits the bladder neck to relax completely to permit bladder emptying. The most commonly prescribed drugs in this category are Proscar and Flomax, respectively. These days you can hardly watch an hour of television without seeing an advertisement for one or another of these drugs. One of the problems with the drug which relaxes the bladder neck is that it can also cause loss of sexual drive and impair ejaculation.

Prostate cancer is the malignant growth of an enlarging prostate. This can usually be diagnosed by manual rectal examination of the prostate by your primary care doctor or by a urologist. Prostate cancer is usually a hardened, irregular area on the prostate. Another test is a blood test for the PSA antigen. If elevated above 3 or 4 ng per milliliter of blood, it is indicative of prostate cancer.

There are a number of available treatments for prostate cancer, all of them with significant drawbacks. One is biopsy of the suspect area of the prostate followed by surgical excision. This can result in impotency as well as greater or lesser incontinence following surgery. Another is to inhibit the growth of the tumor by radiation or cryogenic therapy, that is, freezing the tumor to death. It will be the task for the urological surgeon or oncologist to decide treatment with the patient. Untreated, cancer of the prostate can spread to the bones or nearby organs, such as the bladder or the rectum. One other approach to cancer of the prostate is to bank on the fact that most prostate cancers grow only very slowly, and in some cases it may be assumed that the patient who is already of advanced age would live no longer for other reasons and that the cancer will have no impact on his longevity. This is of course a calculated risk which cannot be precisely quantified. But if one wants to assume the risk, the treatment of choice may be to do nothing.

Polymyalgia Rheumatica (PMR)

This complicated-sounding disorder is actually one of the most perplexing disorders to occur in older people. It is not always easy to recognize and diagnose because of its somewhat confusing symptoms and because it is relatively uncommon. It is characterized by sudden onset of severe muscle and joint stiffness and pain, weight loss, fatigue, and low-grade fever, along with loss of appetite and actual muscle wasting. These symptoms occur because of a destructive immune system reaction of muscles based on inflammation of the arteries supplying those muscles. There are specific tests that indicate whether there is in fact inflammation of muscle tissue. These include elevation of the erythrocyte sedimentation rate (ESR) and elevation of an inflammatory indicator, called C-reactive protein. Once recognized, however, the condition responds very well to treatment, which consists of the anti-inflammatory agent, prednisone. A rapid, positive response to anti-inflammatory corticosteroid therapy is in fact confirmation of the diagnosis. Initially quite high doses may be needed. This should be gradually reduced, and eventually discontinued. Very lengthy treatment or failure to discontinue the prednisone treatment may lead to demineralization of bone, particularly bones of the spine, which can then lead to vertebral fracture, a very painful condition. Also, lengthy treatment with prednisone or similar steroidal anti-inflammatory medication can also lead to bleeding ulcers of the stomach. If the treatment needs to be continued for more than a few weeks, bone-rebuilding medications such as Fosamax, Actonel, or Boniva may be indicated. Also indicated to prevent ulcer formation may be medications that reduce stomach acid formation such as Nexium or Prilosec.

Replacement Surgery

All of our parts do not seem to wear out at the same time. For this reason, and because of advances in the field of medical devices and equipment, it is now possible to replace worn-out parts somewhat like we do brakes or tires on our automobile. Knee replacement, hip replacement, and even shoulder replacements, are now quite possible and are becoming more commonplace. These involve primarily the replacement of skeletal parts, largely simple joints, like those at knee, hip, and shoulder. They can be replaced surgically by specific manufactured mechanical devices. Replacement of organs that require new tissue growth, such as heart, lung, or liver transplants, are discussed in another section of this appendix. I talked earlier about replacement of lenses of the eye to replace lenses that had become opalescent due to cataract formations.

Respite Care

Respite care is an interesting type of service in that it can imply respite for both the patient and the caregiver. Respite care might include an adult daycare service for someone with Alzheimer's disease. On the one hand, the caregivers experience respite or a reprieve from their caregiver responsibilities, allowing them time for themselves to attend to personal needs or desired leisure activities. Patients attending adult daycare services, on the other hand, may also enjoy a respite from their routine activities to socialize and participate with others in activities that they might particularly enjoy, such as listening to music or dancing, or guided reminiscence provided at the daycare center. Another type of respite care is when someone like a patient with Alzheimer's disease is temporarily admitted to an assisted living facility or a memory disorder unit in a nursing home while the caregiver attends some necessary or even enjoyable function, such as participating in a child's graduation or wedding, or just takes a well-deserved vacation. Here the benefit goes primarily to the caregiver, while the patient placed in respite care may be perfectly okay, but probably would not regard this as an improvement in his or her situation.

Sleep Apnea

Sleep apnea is a serious condition in which normal breathing during sleep is interrupted for extended periods of time, followed by deep respirations. The effect is poor rest and may include daytime sleepiness and decreased intellectual functioning. It can best be diagnosed by a sleep study in a sleep laboratory. If confirmed, it can be treated by positive pressure oxygen administration during nighttime sleep, and sometimes it can be benefited by medications such as Provigil or Nuvigil.

Skin Cancers

Skin cancers are common in older persons. They occur as a result of exposure to sunlight during earlier years. Both squamous cell carcinoma and basal cell carcinomas are common. While these conditions are technically cancers, they are non-invasive and can be treated by a simple surgical procedure in the office of a dermatologist. Melanomas, however, are true cancers; they are invasive and can metastasize. They need to be followed closely for possible recurrence. Melanomas are often irregular in shape, may contain melanin, a black pigment, and may bleed easily. Melanomas are probably also related to excessive exposure to sunlight, but many melanomas are on the palms of hands and soles of feet, which are not exposed to the sun.

Spinal Stenosis

Spinal stenosis, or a narrowing of the spinal canal, is a common cause of backache in persons in their 60s, 70s, and 80s. It requires thorough evaluation to see whether exercise or yoga can alleviate the problem or whether neurosurgical intervention is necessary. Since the condition can seriously limit the activities of those affected, remediation should definitely be sought.

Support Groups

I had previously discussed the value of support groups for caregivers of Alzheimer's patients. But support groups can be highly beneficial for those affected by a number of other diseases, such as arthritis, breast cancer, prostate cancer, or similar conditions. By participating in such groups individuals can learn information and coping techniques related to their particular malady or condition.

Tai Chi

Tai chi is another method for reducing stress. Originally developed in China as a method of self-defense, it has also been described as "meditation in motion." Tai chi involves a series of movements and postures performed in a slow, dance-like fashion. I have enjoyed seeing tai chi exercise performed in a number of public parks near Chinatown in San Francisco, and have always enjoyed the beatific smiles on the faces of participants young or old. Just watching the activity has given me peace, but more is to be gained from participating in the activity than from watching it. There are a number of excellent DVDs available that can teach you to perform tai chi movements. While beneficial whenever tai chi is performed, it is most valuable as a communal activity. I could become virtually rhapsodic about the elegance and beauty of tai chi movements.

Testamentary Capacity

Testamentary capacity defines whether an individual is mentally capable of making a valid will. In order to do so, the person must be able to understand that they are making a will, understand the property that they can leave to others in their will, and understand the "natural objects of their bounty," that is, whatever family and friends the individual has, as well as the nature of any organization that they might wish to mention in their will. The concept of testamentary capacity also incorporates the idea that the decision is made freely and without coercion or undue influence. Testamentary capacity is sometimes contested in individuals who are affected by Alzheimer's disease or other forms of memory problems. For this reason making or changing a will should occur very early in patients with Alzheimer's.

Vitamins, Minerals, Hormones, and Other Supplements

The available information about vitamins, minerals, hormones, and other supplements can be both confusing and overwhelming. Because this area of health care is not strictly regulated by anyone, commercial exploitation of vulnerable populations such as the elderly can be as much a motivating factor as is trying to provide a real health benefit. So buyer beware!

Having said that, there is nevertheless a great deal of value in this category of health-related products. It has been clearly established that a minimum of certain vitamins and minerals is necessary for healthy nutrition and normal bodily functioning at all ages. Most once-a-day multivitamins, especially those labeled "for seniors," provide the majority of vitamins and minerals that you as a person in retirement will need if you eat a relatively diverse diet and are not suffering from major medical problems that impact nutrition. The difference between senior and regular once-daily vitamins is the fact that senior vitamins do not contain significant amounts of iron, as iron replacement is no longer needed after the cessation of menstruation with its monthly blood loss. So I recommend that starting at age 60 or 65 both men and women begin to take one senior vitamin tablet or capsule daily. In addition, the Department of Agriculture mandates the addition of numerous B vitamins and folic acid in virtually every product produced from grains, whether that be bread, pasta, cookies, or breakfast cereal. So most of you will not need to take additional B vitamins or folic acid. If you have a documented vitamin B12 deficiency associated with a low blood count or anemia, injections of vitamin B12 should be prescribed by your primary care doctor.

As to hormones, especially sex hormones such as estrogen and progesterone, the information is quite

confusing. There is evidence that estrogen, taken together with progesterone, and taken over a period of
one to three years after the start of menopause, may
have distinct health benefits. Continuing beyond that
length of time has been associated with either no benefit or the possibility of a greater risk for breast cancer,
and is currently not recommended. For a time estrogen compounds were also thought to benefit patients
with Alzheimer's disease. This idea has now been dis-
credited: Not only is there no benefit as far as memory
is concerned, but a significant side effect of estrogen
therapy can be deep vein thrombosis, which is associated with both severe leg pain and the risk of pulmonary embolism, which can be fatal. The only currently
recommended use of estrogen today is in the form of an
estrogen cream applied locally to the vaginal area to improve vaginal texture and lubrication. See chapter 13,
on maintaining your sexuality.

Other vitamins, such as high doses of vitamin A, C,
and E have also been touted at times to be beneficial,
but the data are either confusing or contradictory, and
I cannot recommend that any of these be taken in high
doses other than the doses contained in daily multivitamins. Don't be surprised, though, if you hear con-

trary opinions expressed in social circles, in newspaper health columns, or on TV, especially in TV commercials. Most of all, be sure to let your primary care physician know what vitamins, minerals, hormones, and other supplements you are taking, and ask his or her advice on the topic.

Wheelchairs, Walkers, Quad Canes

If you or your spouse come to be in need of a wheelchair, a walker, or a supportive cane, it is important that you chose the safest and most comfortable assistive device available. In terms of a wheelchair, you should consider a motorized version, or a scooter. When prescribed for you by your physician, this should be no more costly than a standard wheelchair, and in fact its cost may be covered completely by Medicare. The same may be true when acquiring a walker or an assistive cane. Walkers should be lightweight, collapsible for easy transportation in a car, and have wheels to allow the person to propel himself or herself forward. I sometimes refer to the fancier type of walker as the person's "Cadillac," or more recently, as their "Lexus." This usually draws a smile from the "driver." For support, quad canes are probably best, since they can provide the greatest amount of stability. Again, cost should not be the determining fact. A fall or other avoidable injury would be far more costly, in many ways, than the purchase of the safest, best-designed assistive device.

Yoga

Yoga is a form of exercise combined with deliberate attention to breathing. It consists of a number of poses or positions designed to increase strength and flexibility. These poses can range from lying on the floor in a completely relaxed position to assuming a number of complex poses that require considerable strength, balance, and flexibility. Originated in India, it began as a philosophical as well as a mental and physical health strategy; it is now widely practiced in western society as well. Yoga is a mind-body type of medical intervention used primarily for stress reduction, but it can also be beneficial in the treatment of back conditions such as lower back pain. You will need to join a yoga class and be taught by a yoga instructor. To some degree yoga lessons can also be learned from DVDs on yoga. The relaxation, flexibility, and strength benefits that yoga provides are generally added to traditional medical treatments and medications. Again, under close supervision, yoga is a side-effect free strategy with many benefits. However, it must be done under appropriate supervision in order not to stress muscles and joints until sufficient balance and strength have been built up.

Zoster

Shingles, a disease caused by the herpes zoster virus, produces painful inflammation of nerves of the chest, back, or face. It occurs most commonly in older persons. It can last for several weeks or even months, and may leave residual pain along the track of the inflamed nerves. This is called post-herpetic neuropathy. Shingles can be treated in its early stages with antiviral medication. The best technique, however, is to prevent shingles by a single vaccination which has now been developed, and which should be administered to most or all older persons by their primary care physician.

List of Resources

Here is a list of additional resources that you may wish to consult regarding a specific illness, condition, or helpful agency relevant to an age-related problem. This list is by no means exhaustive, so if you do not find a specific topic or organization here, you may wish to turn to one of the major internet-based search engines such as Google or Bing, for instance.

Alzheimer's Association

The Alzheimer's Association is the largest advocacy organization in support of individuals affected by Alzheimer's disease. It provides information about diagnostic and treatment services, caregiver support services, description of the disease, and other issues. The organization has a significant lobbying arm that seeks to influence legislation related to Alzheimer's disease research and services. It has chapters in virtually every major community throughout the United States. You can locate the one in your community by calling 1-800-272-3900 or finding it on the Internet under www.alz.org. Each regional Alzheimer's Association chapter also lists affiliated Alzheimer's caregiver support groups on a county by county basis.

American Association of Retired Persons (AARP)

The American Association of Retired Persons (AARP) is the largest membership organization advocating for older persons in the United States. It has a significant lobbying arm that seeks to influence legislation affecting older persons. Membership is open to all persons over age 50. AARP also has a number of other programs, including the magazine, *AARP*, an insurance program, and various discount programs favoring older people. You may call AARP at 1-800-OUR-AARP or find it on the internet under http://www.aarp.org.

Area Agencies on Aging

Area Agencies on Aging are federally funded community organizations designed to assist elderly persons in finding health, social, respite, and other services. They can also help you find volunteer opportunities, meal service sites, and senior centers as well as respite care programs. Every sizeable community has one or is served by one. They can be found in your local phone books under a listing of federal government agencies, or through the national Eldercare Locator (see below).

Eldercare Locator

The Eldercare Locator is a public service provided by the Administration on Aging of the United States government. It provides a listing of all Area Agencies on Aging as well as all State Units on Aging. Through your local Area Agency on Aging you can find access to community health care, nutrition, home care, and caregiver services. Call 1–800–677–1116 or find it on the Internet under http://www.eldercare.gov.

Meals On Wheels

Meals On Wheels is another community service available to older people who can no longer regularly cook for themselves. Meals On Wheels can help prevent malnutrition, but in addition it will bring you much-needed social contacts. Meals On Wheels is available at little or no cost for people who need this service. Delivering meals can be a rewarding volunteer activity for those who are still mobile and wish to serve others. The social relationships that sometimes develop out of such activities can be remarkably enjoyable. You can find Meals On Wheels programs listed in the white pages of your telephone directory.

Medical Information Websites

One of the best known and probably most trustworthy medical information websites for a broad range of medical information is http://www.WebMD.com. It is a well-organized and well-documented website on which you can look up information on most medical illnesses as well as on medications.

Another useful and well-documented website is the

Mayo Clinic Medical Information Service, which you can find at http://www.MayoClinic.com. The site is organized by medical diseases and conditions, and for each illness it provides a list of symptoms, treatment options or wellness solutions, and general advice to those affected by that disease.

Another medical information service is MedlinePlus, a service provided by the U.S. National Library of Medicine and the National Institutes of Health. It can be reached at http://www.nlm.nih.gov/medlineplus/. Both health care providers and consumers use this service. In Chapter 6, I recommend that you become as familiar as possible with all the medical conditions and medications that relate to your own health status. This is in addition to the advice from your primary care doctor and the specialists to whom you have been referred. This is the best way that you can become your own health care manager.

If these resources are not sufficient to meet your informational needs, you can also enter the specific medical illness or condition and/or the specific medication that you are concerned about in one of the general Internet search engines, such as Google or Bing.

Visiting Nurse Associations

Visiting Nurse Associations operate in virtually every sizeable city in the U.S. They are an excellent source for arranging for home health care services by individuals who are trained and certified to provide outstanding service. In addition, they are non-profit organizations and provide services regardless of ability to pay. Their member nurses are capable of providing complex medical services under the direction of a physician in the patient's home. The services provided by a Visiting Nurse Association compare favorably with those provided by for-profit home health care providers.

Afterword

I want to thank you for reading this book; I am honored that you have chosen to read it. To some degree you have become acquainted with me, and I wish that I could become more acquainted with you. You could write to me at my e-mail address, epfeiffe@health.usf.edu, and tell me something about your retirement experience. You could let me know what parts of the book were meaningful to you and which were not. I'd like to hear from you.

We are all in this together; we are all connected. Throughout history few people have lived as long as you and I, so we are pioneers of a kind.

If I have revealed here a little too much of myself, so be it. I make no apologies. We are all here for only a little while, just passing through. We are human, made of the same stuff.

Index

INDEX

EOBs (Explanation of Benefits Statements), 60–61
EPA (eicosapentaenoic) antioxidants, 134–35
E-readers and e-books, 268
Erectile dysfunction, 206–9, 211–12, 215
Erythrocyte sedimentation rate (ESR), 281
Estrogen and estrogen creams, 210, 212, 289–90
Exelon, 118, 124–25
Exercise: benefits of, 67, 161–62, 171; for brain maintenance, 134; case examples of, 169, 172–73; charting progress in, 166; and different health problems, 84, 86, 88, 252, 256, 264–65, 286; as fun activity, 171–73; goals of, 162–63; overcoming obstacles to, 167; passion for, 170; pedometer for, 76–77, 164; personal trainer for, 168–69; for recovery after illnesses or injuries, 65; reduction of medications with, 171; restarting after period of forced inactivity, 166; rewards for, 172; as social occasion, 167–68; stationary bikes and other exercise machines, 164–65; strength training, 163, 165, 171; walking briskly, 163–64
Explanation of Benefits Statements (EOBs), 60–61
Eye diseases, 263–64, 283

Falls, 135–36, 171, 179, 273, 292
Family members: as caregivers of Alzheimer's patient, 120, 126–30; grandchildren, 37, 49,

50–52; inheritance for, 45–46, 146–49, 287–88; joint checking account with, 182; living with, 21; and parent's decision to live with significant other, 46–47; and parent's remarriage, 45–46; powerful statements to, 245–47; social relationships with adult children, 42. *See also* Spouse/partner
Fasting blood sugar levels, 75
Fibromyalgia, 264–65
Finances: annuities, 142–45; case examples of, 155–58; categories of money, 139–53; charitable remainder trust, 145; from consulting, 29, 150–51; and financial advisor, 159, 225; guaranteed money, 139–46; income level in retirement versus working years, 138–39; income tax reduction, 154–56, 182; investing, 151–52; maintaining financial independence, 182; money that is not guaranteed, but can become inheritance, 140, 146–49; new money or earned income in retirement, 140, 149–53; from part-time or full-time work, 29, 149–50; pensions, 141–42; power of attorney for, 182; principal residence, 148–49; rental property or rental income, 147; royalties on intellectual property, 147; and scams, 156–59; selling on Internet and in consignment stores, 152–53; Social Security, 141, 154; stocks and bonds not in retirement account, 147

305

Financial advisors, 159, 225
Fish oil, 134–35, 265–66
Fixed annuities, 143–45
Flomax, 279–80
Flu (influenza), 82–83
Flu shots, 71, 82
Food. *See* Diet and nutrition
Foot care, 277–78
Forgetfulness. *See* Memory loss
Forgiveness, 226, 242
Fosamax, 274, 282
Fractures, 136, 186, 273
Freedom, 47–48, 195–96
Friendships. *See* Social relationships

Gastrointestinal disorders, 269
Geriatric care managers, 266–67
Gibbons, Leeza, 218
Gift giving, 243–44. *See also* Charitable giving
Glaucoma, 263–64
Glucophage (metformin), 84–85
Glucosamine, 93
Goals, 2–4, 192
Golf carts, 181
Gonorrhea. *See* Sexually transmitted diseases (STDs)
Goodwill, 219
Google. *See* Internet
Grandchildren, 37, 49, 50–52
Gratitude, 237–38, 246
Greenspan, Alan, 7
Grief, 8–9, 43–44, 101–2. *See also* Depression

Hafiz, 197–98
Happiness, 13, 99–100
HDL (high-density cholesterol), 134
Head trauma, 135–36

Health care: for accidents or injuries, 63–64, 135–36; for acute illnesses, 55, 62–63, 136; advocacy corps for, 80–81; avoidance of unnecessary hospitalizations, 65–66; becoming own health care manager, 72; for chronic illnesses, 55, 63; co-manager of, 72–73; complete healing and recovery after illnesses or injuries, 64–65; and concierge medicine, 78–79; diagnostic tests and procedures, 77–78; and electronic medical record (EMR), 80; and Explanation of Benefits Statements (EOBs), 60–61; and geriatric care managers, 266–67; Health Maintenance Organizations (HMOs), 61–62; home health care, 267–68; legal documents for, 182; reducing risk of chronic illnesses, 66–72; Ten Commandments of Wellness, 66–71; and vaccinations, 71; and vital statistics, 73–77; websites on, 297–98. *See also* Health insurance; Illnesses; Medicare; Mental health; Nurses; Physicians; Primary care physicians
Health insurance, 57, 58, 59, 60–61, 108–9
Health Maintenance Organizations (HMOs), 61–62
Hearing loss and hearing aids, 262–63
Heart attack, 87–88
Heart-healthy diet, 67–68, 86, 88
Heart problems. *See specific problems* (such as Congestive heart failure)
Heart rate, 74–75
Helping others, 238, 242

171; undesirable sexual side
effects of, 206–7, 208, 209, 212.
*See also specific illnesses and medi-
cations*
Meditation, 65, 70, 199, 270. *See
also* Inner, spiritual self
Medline-Plus, 298
Melanomas, 285
Memoirs. *See* Autobiography and
memoirs
Memory loss: benign forgetfulness,
115–16; dementia, 121, 127–28;
fear of, 113–14; minor cognitive impairment, 116–18; types
of, 114–28. *See also* Alzheimer's
disease
Mental health, 95–100. *See also*
Mental health problems
Mental health counselors, 111
Mental health problems: active
involvement in treatment of,
109; addiction to pain medications, 106–7, 249–51, 260;
alcohol abuse, 105–6, 121, 136;
anxiety disorders, 104–5, 270;
depression, 8–9, 44, 102–4,
209, 270; health insurance for,
108–9; normal and abnormal
grief reactions, 43–44, 101–2;
treatment of, 107–11
Metabolic syndrome (pre-diabetes),
83–85
Metformin (Glucophage), 84–85
Minerals. *See* Vitamins and minerals
Minor cognitive impairment, 116–18
Money. *See* Finances
Monounsaturated fatty acids
(MUFAs), 271
Morphine, 250
Moses, Grandma, 7

MRI (magnetic resonance imaging),
117–18
MUFAs (monounsaturated fatty
acids), 271
Muscle-building activities, 163, 165,
171
Muscle relaxation. *See* Relaxation
Myocardial infarction (heart
attack), 87–88

Namenda, 124–25
National Institutes of Health, 298
National Library of Medicine, U.S.,
298
Nature, 238–39
Neuropathy, 249, 261, 277
Neuropsychologists, 117–18
Nexium, 282
Nitroglycerin paste or tablets, 88,
208–9
Nurses, 187, 233, 266–68
Nursing homes, 186–87, 215
Nutrition. *See* Diet and nutrition
Nuts, 271
Nuvigil, 285

Obituary, 231
Occupational therapy, 186, 268
Omega-3 fatty acids, 134–35,
265–66
Oncologists, 91–92, 258, 280. *See
also* Cancer
Organ transplants and organ dona-
tion, 272–73
Osteoarthritis, 92–93, 252
Osteoporosis, 273–74
Over-the-counter medications, 136,
250. *See also* Medications
Overweight, 67–68, 84, 86, 169. *See
also* Diet and nutrition

About the Author

Eric Pfeiffer, M.D., is Emeritus Professor of Psychiatry and the founding Director of the Eric Pfeiffer Suncoast Alzheimer's Center at the University of South Florida College of Medicine in Tampa, Florida, and the Vice Chairman of the Board of Directors of the USF Health Byrd Alzheimer's Institute. He has been honored and recognized for his many achievements. In 1977, he was awarded the Allen Gold Medal for outstanding achievement in the area of geriatric psychiatry by the American Geriatrics Society. In 1985, he was honored for his work in the area of Alzheimer's disease through the establishment of the Eric Pfeiffer Chair in Alzheimer's Disease Research at the University of South Florida. Most recently, Dr. Pfeiffer has been nominated for the Senior Living Media Award of the Florida Council on Aging.

Dr. Pfeiffer is the author of *The Art of Caregiving in Alzheimer's Disease*, and he has written and edited numerous major medical textbooks and journal articles. He has also published two books of poetry: *Take with Me Now That Enormous Step* and *Under One Roof.*

George E. Vaillant, M.D., is a psychiatrist and professor at Harvard Medical School and Director of Research for the Department of Psychiatry, Brigham and Women's Hospital.